Advance Praise for *Life* 2.0

"Kevin has not only redefined the world around him but his ability to inspire and motivate others in the path of happiness and faith-filled living is remarkable! His love for family and care for all those who meet him have inspired me to a better version of myself. More people should strive to have the strength and passion that Kevin exemplifies in everyday life; imagine the world if we all rejoiced as Kevin does in 2.0!"

Susan K. Moats, DNP, MBA, RN, NEA-BC
East Region Chief Nursing Officer
Vice President of Patient Care Services

"Kevin Kirksey has transformed a challenging life experience into a lifelong pursuit of 'Wellness' which has been an inspiration to many."

Dr. David Moore, MD
Cardiothoracic Surgeon

"Simply put, Kevin Kirksey squeezes the most out of every day. He sees the world through a different lens now, and Kevin will tell you that wherever he is the view is outstanding."

Mark Valentine
Hospital President

"Kevin is a successful businessman who underwent a momentous, life-changing experience that few will experience. He is a gifted narrator of the extraordinary events he lived. His story will uplift his readers, comfort patients undergoing treatment, and inspire caregivers fulfilling their life's calling. Read this unforgettable story that could change the way you view your own life."

Jennifer Coleman Stribling, M.A.
Healthcare Executive

"I've never met a person as grateful and appreciative of nurses, doctors, and the whole healthcare team as him! Over the years Kevin, and his beautiful wife June, kept in touch. In one of his letters to us, he said that when life gets tough, I should remind myself of the great work I and our system do for our patients. KEVIN in fact stands for Kind, Enthusiastic, Valiant, Inspiring, and Noble. Mother Teresa said, 'It is not how much we do, but how much love we put in the doing. It is not how much we give, but how much love is put in the giving.' I believe Kevin carried this on in writing this book."

Editha Guevara
RN,MSN,AGACNP-BC
Nurse Practitioner, Cardiothoracic Surgery

"It is patients like Kevin Kirksey that make me want to continue my nursing career and help change as many lives as possible. His life-changing event has given him the determination to change the world and make it a better place. Kevin is an inspiration to anyone that gets to hear his wonderful story."

Brandon Driver
RN, BSN Clinical Nurse Supervisor

"Kevin is an inspiration to all who meet him and a great role model for anyone who has experienced a heart event and is ready to make healthy lifestyle changes to get back on the right track."

Julie Dunagan, MS, CCRP, CEP, FAACVPR

"It is nearly impossible to accurately describe what it is like to know K2.0. I had the pleasure of meeting him in cardiac rehab at THHBP, and little did either of us know at the time, he was able to help heal my heart. Kevin is seemingly flawless at sprinkling his selfless love, showing his genuine affinity for the common good, and making an identifiable impact on many hearts and lives."

Kellea Darwin
Former Exercise Physiologist, Cardiac Rehabilitation

"Sometimes Kevin says he's filled with gratitude and thankfulness. Other times, you'll simply see and feel it leaping from his soul"

Randy Johnson, Hospital Marketing Director

Life 2.0

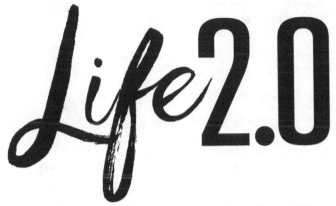

Life 2.0

A Journey from Near Death to New Life

KEVIN KIRKSEY

NEW YORK

LONDON • NASHVILLE • MELBOURNE • VANCOUVER

Life 2.0

A Journey from Near Death to New Life

Published in New York, New York, by Morgan James Publishing. Morgan James is a trademark of Morgan James, LLC. www.MorganJamesPublishing.com

ISBN 9781631950469 paperback
ISBN 9781631950476 eBook
Library of Congress Control Number: 2020933135

Cover & Interior Design by:
Christopher Kirk
www.GFSstudio.com

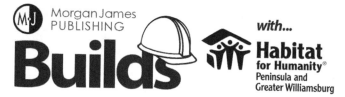

Morgan James is a proud partner of Habitat for Humanity Peninsula and Greater Williamsburg. Partners in building since 2006.

Get involved today! Visit
MorganJamesPublishing.com/giving-back

Table of Contents

Acknowledgments

*M*y wife, June, for her unwavering love, patience, and understanding throughout this journey.

Kevin, Jennifer, and Kevin III for demonstrating the importance and priority of family.

The countless, tireless, and selfless cardiac caregivers and supporting staff at Baylor Scott & White The Heart Hospital – Plano. Not only are you a source of hope and inspiration, but you also unconditionally loved and cared for me during my darkest and scariest times, and, in doing so, made possible the most beautiful blessing of all: Life 2.0.

The American Heart Association for their efforts to raise awareness of the war on cardiac disease and for their support of me helping them with that mission.

Dr. Moore and Dr. Woolbert for saving, restoring, extending, and enhancing my life. Thank you for giving me more time with my family through your medical talents and loving ways.

Randy Johnson for his immense encouragement and support of my speaking and writing efforts to deliver my message and raise awareness and for his confidence in including mine among letters of recommendation for his organization to receive an award.

Dan for being my cardiac rehabilitation buddy and for becoming a close and dear friend during and after our time together at the hospital.

Mark Valentine and Susan Moats for your unrelenting support of me and my family and for the many opportunities you provided for me to express my appreciation and gratitude to your organizations.

Aubrey Kosa, not only for her enormous editing talent but also for her patience and kindness as she guided me through the process of developing a final manuscript, one that came alive because of her creative approach to her work.

David Hancock at Morgan James Publishing for believing in me and inspiring me to work hard and make you proud. The rest of the team at Morgan James Publishing for guiding me through the publishing process, especially Jim Howard and Bonnie Rauch for your support, creativity, passion, and dedication, Bethany Marshall, Publishing Director, and the Author Support Team: Nickcole Watkins, Amber Parrott, and Taylor Chaffer.

All of you impacted by cardiac disease for your efforts to raise awareness so that others' lives can be restored, extended, and even enhanced.

God for demonstrating that He does answer prayers and for the angels who walk among us.

Introduction

*M*y wife, June, and I are living in Farmers Branch, Texas, a beautiful community filled with parks, recreation, and amenities for everyone from children to senior citizens. We are about to celebrate our thirty-fourth wedding anniversary. I am fifty-seven and feel on the top of the world. Our son, Kevin Jr., and his wife, Jennifer, are happy and immersed in their careers, and they live just a few miles from us.

June is my life. She is the most beautiful woman I have ever laid eyes on, even more beautiful with each passing year. She is my rock, my voice of reason, and my bringer of solutions to any issue or problem I face. She shows her love and devotion through her service. She never puts her needs or wants ahead of anyone else's, including those of strangers. She is unusually gracious to people;

she is a bright light to everyone who encounters her. I am eternally grateful to have an opportunity to know her, love her, and be her friend; she is the highest priority in my life.

With so much going for me, I feel invincible.

I have no health concerns, symptoms, or issues of any kind. I feel great about how life is going.

Little do I know this is the calm before the storm. This storm is analogous to a category five hurricane heading straight toward me, on the verge of killing me and leaving my family crippled financially and emotionally.

I believe, by the grace of God, I am alive today and living what I have coined "Life 2.0" because of the story you are about to read, beginning with the most crucial question I have ever asked—the question that saves my life.

Chapter 1:

The question that saves my life

I'm one of those people who believe health problems happen to 'the other guy.'

It is Thursday. I have a routine doctor's appointment with my primary care physician of thirteen years, Dr. Stack. He is an excellent doctor and an exceptional human being. I enjoy being his patient, even though he sternly urges me to make healthier choices at these appointments. I have no reason to think my health is in imminent danger, but I try to heed his urging nonetheless.

Fighting rush-hour traffic, I manage to make it to the check-in station in the nick of time. I don't like being late for anything, and because of the heavy morning traffic, I feel a little stressed.

Soon after I check in, I hear a door open and a familiar voice says, "Kevin, come on back."

That familiar voice belongs to Kathy, Dr. Stack's medical assistant. They have been a team for as long as I can remember. The first step is to measure my weight. I always empty my pockets and take off my shoes to get a lower reading on the scale, which never seems to work. As we head to the examination room, I tease her and let her know it is okay with me if she deducts ten or fifteen pounds before she charts my weight. She proceeds to tell me, "It's going to be all right; Doc is in a good mood today."

She says this every time I see her.

Some say I have a big personality. I am outgoing and rarely miss a chance to say hello to people, whether I know them or not. On the way to the examination room, we pass the nurses' station, where I usually see other physicians and their nurses working. I invariably say out loud, "Good morning, everyone!" I usually get a smile from the people in the area. Most of the time, I will even catch a smile escaping Dr. Stack while at his computer, a smile that appears to say, "Looks like Kevin is here."

That day is a busy one for me at work. I am anxious, hoping to have a short visit with the doctor and leave as soon as I can. My routine throughout the years has been to see him, go to the lab for bloodwork, then head right to work.

Once we're in the examination room, Kathy goes about her routine of asking me how I am feeling, confirming my meds are correct, taking my blood pressure, and checking my heart rate. We always chitchat about our lives. She is a pleasant person to be around, as well as an excellent medical assistant.

Soon after Kathy leaves the room, I hear the familiar three knocks at the door and in walks Dr. Stack. He says hello, shakes my hand, and, with his usual friendly smile, asks me how everything's going and how I am feeling. After listening to my lungs and heart, he tests the reflexes in my knees, followed by the pinprick test on the bottoms of my feet. The pinprick test helps determine if I have any neuropathy caused by the type 2 adult-onset diabetes. I often prank him by jerking my leg away in unison letting out a yelp. My reaction to the pinprick test always startles him. Then he chuckles when he learns I am kidding. But today I don't do that because I am in a rush. After asking me if I am getting up in the night to use the restroom, Dr. Stack confirms which of my medications need refills and then gives me his usual lecture instructing me to lose weight and exercise. He always expresses faith and confidence that someday I will take him seriously and change my ways. He saw me do it five years ago when I lost a significant amount of weight, which improved my cholesterol, blood pressure, and blood sugars. I need to make better choices. After all, Dr. Stack informs me that if my sugar levels do not improve, I must start taking insulin. I do not want any part of that.

I shake his hand, thank him, tell him he looks great and to be sure and take care until next time. He reminds me to stop by the lab to have blood drawn before leaving the building, something I do after every visit. In a day or two, I will get a note from Dr. Stack sharing the results of the bloodwork along with his opinion of my health and, of course, encouragement to improve my diet and exercise.

At last, another day with Dr. Stack is complete. As I am leaving the examination room, I stop, turn to Dr. Stack, and out of my mouth comes, "Hey, Doc, I have a question…. I hope this doesn't sound too crazy, because I am feeling great and have no reason to suspect anything is wrong, but is there something on the inside of my body we should check?"

I hear about people spending enormous sums of money doing full-body scans and undergoing a lot of testing to learn more about their health. Even though I don't want to go to that extent, I am curious about what he thinks I should consider doing, if anything at all. In this moment, between me asking the question and him responding, I wonder why I even asked this question. It has not been occupying my mind at all. It just surfaced. I have no reason to suspect anything is wrong. I feel fantastic…perhaps I am curious to learn whether feeling great is really the whole picture.

But Dr.Stack's reaction does not make me think I've asked a silly question. The expression on his face sobers, much more than the rest of the appointment. He thinks for a bit, and then answers matter-of-factly, "You should probably have a coronary calcium scan performed." Even though I feel fine, I do have some risk factors for coronary artery disease, including high blood pressure, high cholesterol, type 2 diabetes, and some family history of heart problems. I am overweight, work a stressful job, and have a history of smoking. I ask him to explain what this test does, how it works, and what I might experience by taking it. I certainly do not want anything invasive, especially when my heart is at stake. He explains that the scan is an imaging test to better understand someone's risk for coronary artery disease. Often the test is ordered for patients who don't have symptoms but have a family history or other risk factors. He proceeds to tell me the test measures the amount of calcium buildup in and around the cardiovascular system; it is not conclusive but is considered a marker test that can identify the need for more investigation. According to Dr. Stack, I should be okay if I have a low score, and, if not, we will deal with that then. He makes me feel comfortable with it, explaining that it is inexpensive and lasts only about ten minutes. He tells me I will lie down, and a machine will measure the amount of calcium buildup throughout my cardiac arteries. A low score is good, a high score warrants further testing. It is that simple.

After I thank him for the recommendation, Dr. Stack informs me this test is performed in the x-ray lab just down the hall. I shake his hand and excuse myself to venture into the rest of my day.

Even though I am in a rush, I find myself curious about this calcium scan. For reasons I can't explain, I decide to stop by the x-ray lab on my way out. After all, it is just down the hall. A simple inquiry won't hurt. A young lady at the check-in desk greets me and asks what time my appointment is. I explain I do not have an appointment, but my doctor suggested I have a coronary calcium scan done and I was looking to see if I was in the right place. She confirms I am and asks my name and date of birth so she can look me up in their computer system. She tells me, "Yes, I see you right here, and if you like we can do the scan right now. It will just take a few minutes."

I'm not sure what to say. The idea of doing the test so soon hadn't occurred to me, and it seems rushed. I let her know I can't do it today due to my workload. She responds, "How about Monday, at 8 a.m.?"

"Sure, put me down," I say somewhat unconvincingly. As I leave, I wonder why I agreed to come back to this facility so soon.

I am happy about taking this step; I feel like I am acting on my health, doing the right thing. I believe the test is just a precaution and will come back with no problems found. It will be $75.00 well spent.

After all, I feel fine.

Chapter 2:

Imminent danger –
1,700 miles from home

*D*uring my drive to work, all I can think about is my interaction with Dr. Stack. Why did I ask the question? Why that one? Why today?

Later that day, June asks how my appointment went. I tell her it was fine, just another routine doctor's visit. I am not sure how she will react to the calcium scan discussion with Dr. Stack, or how the discussion got started, but I share that I have an appointment on Monday to do the scan. June is surprisingly happy to hear this and tells me I am doing the right thing by acting on my health in this way. The very next day is Valentine's Day. June and I celebrate a fabulous dinner at one of our favorite restaurants and enjoy a lovely weekend together.

That Monday, I begin my daily routine of drinking coffee and catching up on some email. Noticing the x-ray lab appointment on my calendar, I begin to wonder whether I should take the time to do the cardiac calcium scan. After all, I have pressing deadlines and a lot of work to do. I am moments away from calling the x-ray lab and canceling. I convince myself I should not be taking time out of my day since I feel fine. But once I realize it is 6:30 a.m. and no one is there to answer the phone, I decide to bite the bullet and go.

If it was an hour later, I would have called and canceled.

While checking in for the scan, I am nervous, most likely due to the unknown factor about what is going to happen. I keep telling myself I am doing the right thing; however, I do not want the machine to find anything wrong.

After all, I feel great.

The technician performing the test is accommodating and provides instructions. What she describes sounds straightforward, and this makes me feel comfortable. All I do is lie down and the high-speed imaging system will take pictures. During the scan, the machine will talk to me, telling me when to inhale and when to exhale. The technician tells me what position to have my body in for each series of pictures. Some are taken while lying on my back, others on my side.

The scans, although precisely like what Dr. Stack and the technician described, seem to take longer than the ten minutes I was expecting. Although there is no way of knowing for sure, I have a sense that parts of the test are being repeated. I am sure it is my imagination at work. When the test finishes, the technician's demeanor seems different than when she first escorted me into the testing area. Again, probably just my imagination.

Slightly nervous about the dynamics in the room due to her possible change in demeanor, I ask, "How did I do?"

She cracks a friendly smile and explains she is not at liberty to tell me anything and my doctor will follow up with me about the results. As we head to the door, I ask if I have calcium buildup, and, if so, is there anything I can do with exercise or diet to reduce it? She tells me the calcium already built up will stay with me for the remainder of my life, and that's all she tells me.

I shake her hand, thank her for doing the scans, and leave the building, thinking how easy those scans were. I am glad it is over, and I look forward to Dr. Stack contacting me with the good news about the results.

Early the next morning—Tuesday—I board a flight from Dallas to San Jose for a business meeting with a customer. I will be joining a colleague of mine, Randy Hunt, for this meeting. Randy and I always work well together, so I am looking forward to the meeting with him and the customer.

The flight is on time; the weather is perfect. After an on-time arrival, I walk to the outside curb of the terminal building. Randy picks me up in his rental car. This day is going very well, as planned. The meeting starts in an hour and a half, so we decide to stop for a cup of coffee and talk for a short while before heading to the meeting.

Our meeting starts on time. Twenty minutes into the meeting, as the discussion with the customer is progressing well, my cell-phone rings. Our session is interrupted; I forgot to turn the ringer off. I apologize to those in the room and immediately send the call to voicemail, noticing a familiar number on the caller ID. After setting my phone to vibrate to avoid another interruption, it takes me a few minutes to realize the phone number on the caller ID is

Dr. Stack's main office number. I think, "What excellent service they give, probably just calling to tell me that the results of the test were excellent."

Ten minutes later, I feel the vibration of my phone, which is now in my pocket. I think, "My goodness, who is calling me now?" Somewhat irritated, I quickly glance to see who is calling me…. It is Dr. Stack's office again. Believing the second call is just a mistake on their part, I send my phone to voicemail again. The third time they call, approximately another ten minutes later, raises my concern. Someone is trying to reach me for sure.

I excuse myself from the meeting and step into the hallway, closing the door behind me so as not to disturb anyone. As I wait for someone to answer the phone, I feel a surge of anxiety. After a few rings, I am greeted by the office receptionist. I tell her my name, explaining that I am out of town on business and someone from their office has called me three times within thirty minutes. I ask if she can find out who wants to speak with me and suggest she check with Kathy. Holding on the line seems like an eternity, even though it was less than thirty seconds. "Kevin? How are you?" asks Kathy's familiar voice.

I explain that someone from the office is trying to reach me and has called three times. She informs me that it was her making those calls and apologizes by saying, "I'm so sorry, Kevin. The results of the test are not good."

"What do you mean, Kathy?" I quickly reply.

She follows by saying, "The scores are the worst that Dr. Stack has ever seen."

Have you ever talked with someone on the phone and had the sense they might be in tears? Kathy seems to be tearing up, although I do not know for sure. Again, I ask, with a more aggressive crescendo in my voice, "What does that mean?"

Her response stuns me: "It means you are at extreme risk of having a cardiac event or stroke at any moment."

Does she mean I could die at any time? What does she mean "at any moment"? The news shocks me; I am not able to process what I am hearing. How can I be on the verge of collapse? I feel great. I am full of energy and exhibit no symptoms whatsoever. "What do I do?" I asked, the only thing I could murmur on the phone. She asks where I am. When I tell her I am in California, she pauses before saying in an eerily calm voice, "Okay, I need you to be calm and come home immediately. Can you come home today? We have made arrangements for you to see a cardiologist."

After another brief pause, I heard Kathy say, "I'm so sorry, baby." After I explain there is no way to get back to Dallas in time for the cardiologist appointment, I let her know I will make every attempt to get back to Dallas that evening. I then ask for her help moving the cardiologist appointment to the next morning. She assures me she will talk care of it, and we say goodbye to one another.

I am so shocked I do not even think to ask her what my score is, why it is considered high, which cardiologist am I seeing, or where I go at what time. I rejoin the meeting and say nothing else because my mind is spinning. Over and over I try to process the risk level Kathy describes and find it impossible. How can I internalize being 1,700 miles from home, feeling great, but knowing the medical equipment is alarmingly reporting that something is seriously wrong with me? Am I about to die? The impact of realizing there is a silent and deadly threat at play is nothing short of surreal. This is something that happens to someone else, not me. I think, "My next step could be my last. I may never see June or my son again." I am overwhelmed with loneliness, helplessness, and fear, having just learned I could drop at any moment while being far away from home.

When the meeting adjourns, I shake hands with our customer, and when we leave the conference room, I pull Randy aside and tell him I have a problem. Once outside, Randy listens to me describe the phone call with Kathy and asks if there is anything he can do. I tell him, "Drive me back to the airport now." Twenty minutes later, Randy drops me off at the curb of the airport terminal. I worry that I might have a heart attack on my way to the ticket counter. My mind must be playing tricks on me. I have never encountered a situation where I'm told something terrible might happen at any moment— to me. I arrive at the counter and look the agent in the eyes, very calmly saying, "I just flew in two hours ago. I now have a medical emergency, and I need your help to get me back to Dallas as soon as possible please." Without saying another word, I hand her my credit card. I can see compassion in her eyes; she goes to work and immediately confirms me on a flight that leaves in two hours and does not charge me any fare difference or change fees. She smiles, saying, "I hope you are well. Good luck."

I call June to let her know I arrived, something I always do when I travel. I decide not to let her know I am coming back home. Shortly after June answers the phone, I learn that her friend, Lois, is visiting. June and Lois enjoy laughter and watching old movies together. I do not want to disturb her time with Lois with my news, so I lie and tell her I am just calling to say hello. Wishing her an enjoyable time with Lois and letting her know I will check in with her later, I hang up. I am not the least bit hungry, but to pass the time as I wait for my flight home, I sit down at a restaurant table just inside the security checkpoint. I look at people in the restaurant; they all seem happy, carefree, and relaxed. Here I sit, wondering if I am a dead man. I do my best to eat a chicken caesar salad and then head to the gate. As the time to board draws near, I decide to call June again. Lois has just left. I explain the poor test results and that I need to return home to see a cardiologist the next day. "Everything is going to be fine," I tell her with the most reassuring voice I can manage. I explain that I should come home as a precaution only. She expresses her worry about my job and asks if my departing early will hurt our business. I ease her concern by informing her that Randy will be just fine without me during the balance of the trip. June is always so supportive of my career. I promise her everything is okay and tell her I will be walking in the door around 11 p.m. I end our conversation by saying, "Do not worry about anything, honey. I love you. See you soon."

Once on the flight, I learn the plane has Wi-Fi available. I think, "Great, a chance to do some research while traveling home and get a better understanding of what Kathy reported earlier about my calcium scan results." Once in the air, I connect to Wi-Fi and send an email to June informing her the plane is in the air and on the way to Dallas. Naturally, when she receives the email, she knows I am online and available. She replies with, "Tell me again the name of the test you took and exactly what Kathy said."

"Oh boy," I think. That is a strong indication June will also be spending her evening trying to understand what is going on with me. I know how she is.

I frantically search the internet for information about the test while doing my best to comfort June as we send email notes back and forth. My anxiety is at an all-time high from the many "what if" questions my mind conjures up, further complicated by self-conjecture about what might be going on with my health. I am a mess at this point.

I locate a lot of information about the test. Dr. Stack is right; it is just a marker test. It is not conclusive by itself and can serve as a recommendation for further testing. I come across a chart that provides meaning for ranges of scores. A score of 0 means there is no evidence of coronary artery disease, while the highest score I see listed, anything over 400, indicates the possibility of extensive coronary artery disease. The scores in between 0 and 400 range from minimal to moderate evidence of coronary artery disease.

June and I discover this chart at the same time. She sends a copy to me, not realizing I, too, had found it. But in my confusion and shock during the brief conversation with Kathy, I forgot to ask what my score was. I had no idea a score is just a number. After letting June know I forgot to ask Kathy for my score, I write: "There was no way mine was 400 or greater. That is as high as the chart goes." I also realize my score will probably not be low, based on what Kathy said about Dr. Stack's reaction. I try to rationalize my situation as being less severe than I first thought. Just because mine is the worst score Dr. Stack has seen does not mean it is high compared to what cardiologists have seen. I am sure cardiologists see results like mine every day.

I make it home. Neither June nor I can sleep. The anticipation and anxiety are extremely high for both of us. We lie in bed until after 2:30 a.m., thinking and talking about the situation in which we find ourselves. It feels comforting for us, being together at home. Somehow our togetherness eases the anxiety…a little bit.

Chapter 3:

Test score – Need to move fast

The next morning—Wednesday—I have feelings of anxiety and unrest. Before driving to meet with the cardiologist, I call Kathy to find out what my calcium scan score is. Both June and I want to know why their level of concern was so high. Thank goodness Kathy is in the office, and the receptionist tells me she will be with me momentarily. Once Kathy comes to the phone, I thank her for making the arrangements for me to see the cardiologist, which will be within the hour, and I ask about the test result. She asks me to hold for a minute while she retrieves the information. While waiting for her, I am hoping for something less than 100.

I have printed the results chart from the internet so that I have something to compare my results to, providing me with a clue about the severity of my condition.

Kathy returns to the phone to read the results to me. I was right. I did not have a low score, and I also did not have a score of 400. She tells me the composite score is 6,518.

Oh my goodness, something is wrong. How can this be? I can't understand how my score is off the chart when I feel so good. I ask her if Dr. Stack thinks the machine produced a faulty reading. Her reply stuns me, "Kevin, the technician could not believe the results either, especially since the test equipment was calibrated recently, so she ran the test a total of three times and got the same result each time."

I then ask Kathy if she is sure this is my score, and she replies, "Yes, Kevin, I am certain. Sorry to have to tell you this."

This result is approximately sixteen times higher than the highest portion of the internet chart, which implies extensive evidence of coronary artery disease.

I thank her, hang up the phone, and tell June what I just learned. It turns out that, after all, it was not in my imagination that the test took longer than I expected. I had no idea the technician ran it three times. June, too, is in disbelief as the words "oh no" escape her mouth while she looks at me with an expression of despair and helplessness.

My precise results, shown below, break down the scores of each main artery to get the composite score of 6,518.

Coronary Calcium Scan: Score = 6,518

1,057	Left Anterior Descending
472	Left Circumflex
4,914	Right Coronary Artery
75	Posterior Descending Artery
6,518	**Composite Score**

During our drive to the heart center in Plano, Texas for my cardiologist appointment, we both remain in disbelief and shock. A score of 6,518 has not been in the realm of possibility in any of our research and discussions. I try to convince myself the cardiologist will be able to put my mind at ease. After all, this is what he deals with every day, right?

As we pull into the heart center parking lot, my anxiety level increases. I feel slightly reserved, withdrawn, and numb. I have never been to see a cardiologist and have no idea what to expect. I am still unable to comprehend why the medical devices are reporting I am in grave danger while I feel great.

My mind is racing as I wait. Looking around the waiting room, I observe that I am one of the youngest patients there, which frightens me, as I think to myself that I am too young to have serious heart issues.

I wonder if I will collapse before I see the doctor, and, if I do, will they be able to help me?

Thankfully, the cardiologist has a demeanor I find quite calming. My first impression is that he is an astute and articulate physician. I explain the reason for this visit and how I learned this score is the worst my doctor has seen, but, undoubtedly, he deals with this all the time. He immediately shakes his head, replying, "No, I have never seen one this high; we need to start some testing on you immediately."

At this moment, I realize I am in trouble.

He sends me to the scheduling department, where I meet Rochon. I take a seat while Rochon accesses the scheduling system. Having no clue what tests I am going to have performed, I wait quietly and patiently for Rochon to tell me what the plan is. She is searching for some open appointment slots and begins to tell me how full the schedule is. She knows this is important and continues to search for a way to get me in. I look Rochon in the eyes, and I say, "They tell me I am in trouble. I am scared, and I need your help to do whatever you have to do to make this happen as fast as it can. I can't waste time."

I will never forget the compassionate, understanding, and loving look she gives me, replying, "Don't you worry, Mr. Kirksey. We are going to make this happen, and nothing is going to get in our way. I got your back." Although I will never know for sure, it is highly probable that Rochon jumped the scheduling line for me. Perhaps she sees something in my eyes that gives her determination to get me in—fast. She tells me great news; they can have me start testing right away. I ask Rochon who the scheduling department supervisor is, explaining I want to let them know about her willingness and eagerness to help me.

She tells me, "I am the supervisor, Mr. Kirksey, and no need to thank me; it's what I do."

I will never forget this brief moment with Rochon and how she understood the gravity of needing to act fast and make it happen. I see Rochon from time to time and enjoy her smile and hugs. We both remember and acknowledge that moment; I will forever remain grateful to her.

During the next two days, I undergo a variety of tests. The cardiologist explains that no single test is typically conclusive, but, together, they can accurately portray what is happening with my heart. Below are some of the tests.

Electrocardiogram
Also called an EKG or ECG—to check for signs of heart disease. It's a test that records the electrical activity of your heart through

small electrode patches that a technician attaches to the skin of your chest, arms, and legs. With this test, your doctor will be able to:

- Check your heart rhythm
- See if you have poor blood flow to your heart muscle (this is called ischemia)
- Diagnose a heart attack
- Check on things that are abnormal, such as thickened heart muscle
- Detect if there are significant electrolyte abnormalities, such as high potassium or high or low calcium

Stress echocardiography

An exercise stress echocardiogram (stress echo) is a procedure that combines echocardiography with exercise to evaluate the heart's function at rest and with exertion. Echocardiography is an imaging procedure that creates a picture of the heart's movement, valves, and chambers using high-frequency sound waves that come from a hand-held wand placed on your chest.

Stress myocardial perfusion

A cardiac perfusion test tells your doctor if the muscles of your heart are getting enough blood. It's also known as myocardial perfusion imaging or a nuclear stress test.

All test definitions taken from https://www.webmd.com/.

Even with the testing complete, I still do not know anything about the results or my condition. I ask a nurse if there is anyone around who can help me understand what is going on. After a few moments, the cardiologist in the lab approaches me. I ask if he would be so kind as to tell me what's going on; the anticipation is beginning to overwhelm me.

He tells me none of the tests by themselves are conclusive. However, they have discovered my heart is not getting enough oxygen during times of increased load and exertion. He asks several times, with a curious, rather serious expression on his face, "Are you sure you feel okay?"

I look him in the eyes, responding, "This is a little scary. Do I need to check myself into the heart hospital right now?"

He hesitates, for what seems like an eternity, alarming me even further, then says, "We have made arrangements for you to have a heart catheterization in the morning. Go home tonight, be very calm, and come up to the hospital in the morning."

Again, my mind begins to wander. How do I remain calm with the knowledge that something is seriously wrong with me? What if something happens tonight? How do I console June? While trying to be relax during the drive home, I struggle with a feeling of desperation, a sense of having no way out of this mental and emotional prison I find myself in. June and I try to convince each other I will be okay for the night. Why else would a doctor let me go home? The dynamic in the car is either a dialogue about how we will be calm and get through the evening or utter silence—nothing else

Once home, I do not know what I should be doing. Other than changing clothes, my mind is floods thinking that my next step, breath, or conversation with June could be my last. Intermingled with these thoughts and emotions is a desire to prepare for, and come to terms with, death. As I catch myself on the verge of hyper-ventilating, I somehow begin to realize the priority is to make things right with my Maker—while I can.

Chapter 4:

"Young man, you have saved your own life."

The following morning, I arrive at the heart hospital to undergo the cardiac catheterization procedure. Once again, I experience high anxiety. Once again, it is mostly due to the unknown about what is wrong with me and what this procedure will show. All I know is they are going to insert a long, thin tube called a catheter into an artery in my groin and then thread it into my heart. A contrast dye, visible in x-rays, is injected and, from there, they attempt to determine the cause of my problem. All I can think is, "What happens if they puncture an artery? Or find something they can't repair? Or something worse?" I work hard to keep my face looking calm so I don't alarm June.

I hope the cardiologist will determine that all I need is to be put on medication and that I don't require any invasive type of surgery. I am fully aware that the cardiologist could need to open up my arteries with a stent.

Holding June's hand, I walk into the hospital, locate the admissions department, and take a seat by the check-in counter. A nice-looking young man sits across from us, and he introduces himself. He begins to check me in and complete the necessary paperwork. I can't help but notice how kind and polite he is and how he continually smiles. He must hold the record for smiles, and, to top it off, he has a soothing, calming demeanor about him. Just as we were about to ask him where we should go next, he offers, with a smile, "I am going to escort you, get you acquainted and intro-duced personally." Impressed, I make a mental note of his smiles, kindness, and refreshing demeanor.

He escorts us to the preparation room, where he introduces us to the nurse. As he leaves, he offers his assistance at any time. I change into a hospital gown the nurse provides. I tell June how impressed I am with the people we've met so far. They see people like me every day but manage to make me feel quite extraordinary; I appreciate that.

June and I are alone for a few minutes while we wait for some-one to walk us through the rest of the process. I can see the ner-vousness and fear in her eyes. I am sad because I do not know how to help her.

The nurse re-enters the room and, with a warm smile, informs me she will start the IV. In a few minutes, they will take me to the catheterization laboratory. She asks how I am doing today and if I have any questions for her. I tell her I am a little nervous but doing okay. As she begins the insert the IV, I notice she has a difficult time finding a suitable vein. She must have sensed my anxiety and immediately stops what she is doing, takes my hand in hers, and says:

> *"Let's take our time. Whatever time you need, nothing happens until you are okay and ready. I take pride in doing it right for our guests like you."*

It's amazing how her words put me at ease. Knowing I can do things at my pace reduces my anxiety. I ask her to go ahead and try again. This time, she quickly gets the IV started. She tells me the doctor will be in shortly.

Dr. Woolbert enters the room, wearing a smile as he greets us and introduces himself. I get the sense that this guy is an accomplished and experienced cardiologist. Although he must be a very busy man, he makes us feel like we are unique and the most critical part of his day. He proceeds to explain what he is going to do, how long it should last, and what June can expect regarding wait time and recovery. After confirming that I am ready to go, Dr. Woolbert shakes my hand and, with another smile, says he will see me in a few minutes.

A hospital aide comes into the room and explains we are now going to the catheterization lab for the procedure. I hug June, kiss her, and tell her I love her and will see her soon. She is trying to hide her fear.

When we are just outside of the catheterization lab, we stop. The aide tells me they will get me in just a minute. I lie there, alone, indulging in my thoughts. Naturally, the fear of the unknown begins to overtake my emotions; I want to get up and walk out of there. I'm frightened. I feel a hand on my shoulder.

I look up and see a young man who introduces himself as one of the nurses who will be taking care of me during the procedure. After he asks me to confirm my name, he says, "Okay, Kevin. Are you ready for your sex change operation?"

Startled, I look at him, and we both break into laughter. I immediately rid myself of anxiety and fear. Laughter has a way of curing just about anything, and today was an excellent example of that. As odd as it may sound, what that man said to me is the best thing he could have said. He must have tuned into my anxiety and took a chance at reversing it by asking this shocking question.

To this day, I think back on that moment with sincere appreciation for what he did to help me that morning. Fast-forward and I am speaking to a group of hospital professionals. The president of the hospital is in the audience. As I replay the scenario where the nurse asks me if I am ready for my sex change operation, I see his facial expression of disbelief, almost as if he were embarrassed. I immediately tell the audience that what the nurse asks is the perfect question for me—how it broke the cycle of anxiety and fear and put me in a comfortable and relaxed state. I applaud that nurse's ability to read his patients and deal with them uniquely and personably.

That nurse wheels me into the lab. I feel like I am entering a futuristic science fiction laboratory. Lights, monitors, and equipment I have never seen surround me on all sides, including above me. What a high-tech setup.

Once they get me situated and hooked up to the IV, Dr. Woolbert says, "We are ready when you are." I reply that I am ready and ask what happens next.

A nurse leans over and says, "We are going to relax you by injecting some medicine through your IV." Before I can comprehend what he says, I am very calm, with no anxiety and no fear. I feel like I am floating on a cloud in the sky. I think to myself that the medication must be kicking in because I feel great. My mind tries to capture what goes on around me; I hear voices but not much else. I feel a slight pinch in my inner thigh, thinking that must be the catheter they are inserting. That was easy; it does not hurt. The next thing I know, I ask, "How are we doing?"

Dr. Woolbert replies, "Doing great, Kevin, just getting started."

What seems like just a matter of seconds later, I say, "Hey doc, how's it going?"

The next thing I see is Dr. Woolbert's face right next to mine as he says, "Young man, you have saved your own life. There is nothing I can do for you today. Let's get you back with your wife and discuss your options."

I later learn is that Dr. Woolbert aborted the procedure early when he discovered that three of my main coronary arteries were extremely blocked, also called occluded with percentages of blockage at: 100 percent, 90 percent, and 80 percent.

I was at high risk for a sudden and, most probably, fatal cardiac event.

Often a cardiologist is able to place stents to open up arteries and increase blood flow. In my case, with the severe blockage, that is not an option. My procedure lasts only sixteen minutes since there is nothing they can do at this time.

June seems startled as I am wheeled back into the hospital room, asking what happened and why I have returned so early. I tell

June there isn't anything they can do for me and that Dr. Woolbert will be coming to explain.

Dr. Woolbert comes into the room, this time with a more serious expression on his face than before. He explains that, despite it being so short, the procedure was a success since it identified the cause of my problem.

My cardiac catheterization report summarizes the blockages (stenosis) as:

Left Main	Normal with 0% stenosis
Mid LAD	There was a tubular 80% stenosis
Mid Circumflex	There was a 90% stenosis
Proximal RCA	There was a 100% stenosis

As he is explaining these results, June asks, "If one of my husband's arteries is 100 percent blocked, why is he alive today?"

"That is a great question," he replies. "It is what we physicians call God's work." He goes on to explain that the heart muscle knew it was in trouble and, over time, built new arteries, called collateral arteries, to provide blood supply to the heart in the area the blocked artery serves. Collateral circulation is alternate circulation around a blocked artery or vein via another path, such as nearby minor vessels.

He shows us a video of the procedure he just performed on me, and we get to see these collateral arteries. It amazes me that the heart muscle is capable of doing this. He tells June this is what has kept me alive. Even though these collaterals do not carry as much oxygen to the heart during exertion, it is enough to keep the muscle alive during rest.

Okay, now what?

Dr. Woolbert says I have only one option remaining if I want to survive: coronary bypass surgery.

Although it takes a few seconds for his words to sink in, I develop an overwhelming need to move fast. One never truly knows how they will respond to a life-threatening emergency until it occurs. I did not know, until this moment, if I was a "fight" or "flight" kind of guy when confronted with imminent danger. I have an overwhelming sense that I must act fast.

Almost immediately, while feelings of anxiety and fear consume me, I am flooded with thoughts I have never had before.

> *June is not ready; I must fix this, I can't fix this.*
> *Her world was at stake.*
> *My unborn grandchild won't know me.*
> *Have I played catch with my son for the last time?*
> *How do I make peace with my Maker? What are the steps?*

I can't explain why, or how, but I know I have to act. I must move fast—now. I say to Dr. Woolbert, "Man to man, I need help from you. I do not know where else to go."

"Of course I will help you," he replies.

I thank him for doing the procedure and finding out what is wrong with me. I ask him for two things: 1) help me move on this as fast as the healthcare system will allow; 2) since I know nothing about the local heart surgeons, help me find a "starter." I don't want someone off the bench to do this surgery. It's my way of asking him to help me find a world-class surgeon.

He tells me he understands and excuses himself for a couple of minutes. When he comes back into the room, he says we will move fast and that he also just secured a starter, a world-class surgeon who agreed to operate on me. He tells me Dr. David Moore is his name and that I should call his office because they are expecting to see me. What an amazing man to listen to what I truly need his help with and immediately make the arrangements. In my experiences with physicians, it is rare to meet one with such a high degree of vested interest in the patient.

June is noticeably stunned by this news. Although she tries to be strong and hide her fears, I can tell she is trembling while searching for reassurance that this nightmare will end; however, there is nobody who can provide that. We do not discuss my mortality. She is trying desperately to avoid thoughts of life without me.

To this day, Dr. Woolbert remains my cardiologist, as well as June's. He monitors my heart disease, manages my medications, and always shows his genuine interest in maximizing my chances for extended life. He is like a brother to me. We are truly blessed to know Dr. Woolbert and be under his care. As I often say to others, if there were an all-star team for cardiologists, Dr. Woolbert would be the captain.

Chapter 5:

The surgeon – "I'm going to hurt you."

On the way to my first appointment with Dr. Moore, the cardiac surgeon who will perform my surgery, I am nervous. After all, I have never met a cardiac surgeon, let alone one who was going to discuss how to fix my heart.

Upon shaking hands and greeting one another, I sense that he is calm and peaceful, which complements his soft-spoken and gentle personality. Dr. Moore's specialty is cardiothoracic surgery.

After getting acquainted with June and me, Dr. Moore begins to describe the situation I am in and how he plans to fix it. I learn that the severe blockages in my arteries put me at high risk of a fatal attack in the near future. He explains I will need a triple or quadruple bypass, depending on what he observes during the operation.

Coronary artery bypass surgery restores normal blood flow to the heart by creating a "detour" (bypass) around the blocked artery/ arteries by using a healthy blood vessel called a graft. Grafts usually come from the arteries and veins located in the chest, legs, or arms. The graft creates a new pathway to carry blood to the heart.

Because of the large amount of calcium buildup throughout my coronary arteries, the surgeon is not able to decrease the amount of calcium to normal ranges, nor is there medication available to correct my condition. Dr. Moore's objective is to circumvent the most threatening parts of the buildup. He will use his judgment to determine the most optimal approach that will achieve the best possible outcome.

I learn that after I receive general anesthesia, he will make an eight to ten inch incision in my chest and then cut through my sternum, called a sternotomy, to gain access to the heart. They will give me medicine to stop my heart while a heart-lung bypass machine keeps blood and oxygen moving through the body during surgery. This machine will breathe for me and pump blood through my system so that my heart is stable and motionless while the bypasses are put in place. Dr. Moore draws a picture for me, showing me how he will use my mammary arteries for two of the bypasses and a vein, harvested from my left leg below the knee, for the third bypass. The internal mammary artery (IMA) grafts have been associated with improved survival compared to vein grafts.

When the surgery is complete, Dr. Moore will use wires to close my sternum and stitches to close the chest incision. The operation should take four to five hours, followed by a five to seven day stay in the hospital. Two weeks after surgery, I will begin cardiac rehabilitation, which will be three times a week for twelve weeks.

Although I pay close attention to the steps he will take during surgery, I also ask him to describe what my experience will be with this surgery.

> *"Most people who undergo this surgery come out feeling better; they might be less fatigued, or free of chest pain. They see the real and immediate benefit of the surgery. With you, it's a little different because you are asymptomatic."*

He continues:

> *"I need to tell you something. On Monday, I am going to hurt you."*

"Oh my goodness," I think to myself. "Did he say he is going to hurt me?" He continues:

> *"You are going to survive the surgery, and you will recover just fine. You will wonder why you went through all of this, and the pain that comes with it, and, after recovery, you will feel the same as before the surgery. Your mind will play tricks on you. I need to tell you this so you can cope much better with your post-operation experience."*

I thank him for sharing this knowledge and wisdom. I tell him there is something I want him to know. I start by saying I am at peace with my Maker. If I survive, it will be His will, and if my time is up, He will take me. I tell him, "Dr. Moore, I have thoroughly contemplated my mortality and also realize I have done a terrible thing, and I need your help. I have not prepared my wife for my passing. By working so hard to provide for her and fix everything I can along the way, I have crippled her from being able to function on her own. She can't solve problems with the computer, cellphone, or home maintenance." This realization of the terrible thing I have done saddens me greatly. I take June's hand and hold it while I continue to speak with Dr. Moore. I admit to him that if I die now, it will be catastrophic for her. She has had no chance to prepare for anything. I ask Dr. Moore to bring his A game to the operating room—not for me, but for her. I will never forget what he says to me.

> *"Kevin, I am honored, grateful, and privileged for the trust and faith you are giving me with your life, and, yes, I will bring my A game."*

Most doctors, I imagine, would say that of course they will bring their A game. For Dr. Moore to focus on how honored he is that I trust him with my life is a sign of a remarkable human being. When he says this to me, I realize I have a starter, the right guy, the best surgeon for me.

If I had to pick another top-notch surgeon, I would pick one with extensive experience, an excellent reputation, someone who is skilled, smart, and calm. Right after meeting Dr. Moore, I knew I had that top-notch surgeon. If I were to pick a world-class surgeon, they would have those same attributes, plus they would be caring, sincere, supportive, compassionate, gentle, and humble. Because of what he says to me, I know I have a world-class surgeon, and I do not want anyone besides Dr. Moore to operate on me. I know I am in the caring hands of a great surgeon who is also a fabulous human being.

During the drive home, June and I discuss how delightful and refreshing it was to meet Dr. Moore and how fortunate we are to have him be the surgeon who will fix my heart.

I want to live a long life; this is the only choice I have to do that. I have an experienced and successful cardiac team. I am grateful and blessed.

Chapter 6:
Jim's gift

The magnitude of the emotions and thoughts I faced between the day I met with the surgeon and the day of surgery is overwhelming. Here I am, realizing I have crippled my wife, uncertain how she will cope without me. I have worked very hard to provide for her; I did everything. Now I might leave her to live alone and deal with things she doesn't know how to do because I failed to prepare her. I feel ashamed.

Even though I have come to a place of peace with my mortality, I still have unanswered questions. I am frantic as I search for answers to countless questions: "What's going on with me?" "What will happen to me pre, during, and post-surgery?" "Can I endure this, comfort my family, and suppress my fears all at the same time?" I want to know what I should do, what is going to happen to me, in what sequence, and what my survival odds are. How will my family endure the fear, anxiety, and helplessness that enter our lives?

But the most sobering question of all is: "Have I prepared my wife and family for life without me, or will I leave them financially, emotionally, and spiritually crippled?"

"Have I played catch with my son for the last time?" "Have I made love with my wife for the last time?"

The questions and emotions go on and on.

The day when I am to have open-heart surgery is soon approaching. I am anxious, nervous, and afraid. As much as my family and physicians try to provide a state of calm, nothing seems to help. I want to know what it is like to go through it, my coping mechanism perhaps a need to understand the experience before actually going through it.

I am somewhat desperate. I cannot seem to find what I am seeking. Around 8 p.m., two nights before surgery, I walk across the street and knock on Jim's door. Jim is in his eighties, and he lives alone. His dear wife Patsy passed away a few years ago from Alzheimer's disease.

Jim welcomes me into his house. We make some small talk, and then he invites me to sit down. I tell Jim I need his help. I know I'm at the right place; the look he gives me is so full of compassion, so full of love. I share how anxious I am and how I need to know what this surgery experience is going to be like. He has had a few of them himself.

With a spirit of grace, he answers all of my questions, instilling confidence that I was going to be okay. He is in the moment with me during our entire conversation. He is like a father to me that evening. Jim helps me discover what I want to know. When I walk back home across the street, a sense of serenity consumes me. I think of that evening as a gift from Jim. He gave me the gift of comfort and peace during one of the scariest times of my life. It was not until that evening with Jim that I am confident, knowing what is in store for me.

In my writings, speaking engagements, and travels throughout the U.S., Latin America, and Europe, I have shared the story of that evening with Jim and the gift he gave me. Many more people than most could imagine now know about Jim and the kindness he showed to my family and me.

I do not believe I adequately expressed my thanks to Jim for giving me the gift of comfort and peace during one of the scariest times of my life. He holds a special place in my heart and always will.

In a recent email to me, his daughter, Lois, says, "There are many, many stories of Dad bringing serenity to otherwise tense situations. I'm so glad he could be there for you. I am quite blessed to have had him as my father and to have experienced that calming influence my whole life."

A few years after our pre-surgery talk, I find myself visiting Jim at his hospice bedside. You see, it's his turn to rest now. I tell him I love him and thank him again for helping me in a time of need. He puts his hand on mine and whispers, "I love you too." Jim leaves four children, eight grandchildren, and sixteen great-grandchildren behind. I know he and Patsy are dancing together every day, and they have no more suffering.

So, having met with Jim before my surgery, I direct my attention to my work colleagues. At the time, I am responsible for our company's sales worldwide. I have a large staff of people in my organization, and it is appropriate to inform them about my surgery. I do not want them to see me as frightened or weak, but I want to ask for their prayers at 8 a.m. the day of surgery.

I send the following email to my colleagues around the world in Colombia, the Netherlands, United Kingdom, South Africa, France, Australia, and Malaysia.

To my family salesmen and colleagues,

For years, when asked, I have described myself as a "transparent" person. In the spirit of that, I feel compelled to demonstrate transparency by writing to you today. Another thing which many of you have heard emit from my lips is the notion of always giving customers a choice, and as a result, you will find the path your customer wishes to navigate. I still believe that to be true. I genuinely and sincerely do.

I have experienced that life does not always offer choices, but rather, at times, only one offer is made available. Not too long ago, I was about to leave my doctor's office, but decided, on a whim, to ask him a question. "Doctor, I feel fantastic, I have no issues as you know, but I just want to ask if there is anything I should do to see if internally things are okay." To which he replied, "Sure, I suggest you have a coronary calcium scan." Through a fascinating chain of events, I learned this question ultimately saves my life. I need open-heart surgery, as soon as possible.

So what now? I am now facing a situation without choices; the only offer on the table for longevity in life is cardiac bypass surgery. I have been incredibly lucky and blessed. By accident, I take a test, I get an appointment with the only cardiologist who could see me immediately, one whose "stand out specialty" is diagnostics. From there I happen to get a phenomenal, well-known cardiologist to do my catheterization procedure. And another stroke of good luck is that he called on one of the top, most experienced cardiac surgeons in Dallas to operate. His name is Dr. Moore, who, upon hearing my story, accepts me as a patient. I have told him I have complete faith and trust in his judgment, his abilities, his intuition, and his team.

I have some unfinished business in this world; I am prepared, and I have come to a place of peace with my Maker. My fate is in His hands.

Now that I feel like I have been transparent with all of you, and since all good salesmen ask questions, I have one for you. They say this surgery, on average, will require a 5-7 day stay in the hospital, then recovery and therapy. I have never gone that long disconnected from the company I work for. Even when I vacation I don't ignore my work, so this is going to be very difficult for me, but again I don't have choices this time, just the one offer. My question is, will you help me out by taking care of business while I am away? My wish for each of you is to make things happen, go above and beyond, and be your personal best.

Michael is intimately in tune with the details of what I am facing, and please know that he and the rest of the executive team are there to help plug any gaps and holes during my time away.

I love this company and all of you, so thank you for all that you do and who you are. The surgery begins around 8 a.m.. I am grateful for any prayers at that time.

Below are some examples of the kind, compassionate, and loving comments I received from my colleagues.

"Never underestimate the heart of a champion, we're all behind you, Kevin." – Brendan (Canada)

"Words cannot adequately express our respect and love for you as a friend and leader. We are all praying for a successful procedure, a speedy recovery, and a quick return to your work family. You were born to lead." – Ken (Texas)

"We will pray for you and Dr. Moore. The Lord is in control now; nothing is too big for Him. He will send you an Angel. I will begin my prayer at 8 a.m. Texas time. I am looking forward to you visiting my home and giving me the privilege to make you dinner.

This verse was put on my heart to give to you and your family. Spoken by Jesus: Peace I leave with you, my peace I give unto you: not as the world giveth, give I unto you. Let, nor your heart be troubled, neither let it be afraid – John 14:27

All will be well. Your heart will be healed physically and spiritually." – Pieter (South Africa)

"You're a beautiful human being whom I have grown to love and appreciate. Know for sure you will get through this better and stronger than ever. God Bless you, and I will be praying for you at 8 a.m." – Bill (Massachusetts)

"I want to share this old Celtic blessing.

May the road rise to meet you,
May the wind be always at your back.
May the sun shine warm upon your face,
The rains fall soft upon your fields.
And until we meet again,
May God hold you in the palm of his hand.
May God be with you and bless you,
May you see your children's children.
May you be poor in misfortune,
Rich is blessings.
May you know nothing but happiness
From this day forward.
Hugs," – Anderson (Columbia)

"I am not sure if I should feel sad about this or happy about the fact that you found out in time. I am sure

with your strong character; you will walk out of this even stronger. My thoughts and prayer are with you and your family. I cannot wait to have you back. God Bless." – Shahab (Canada)

"Our blessings and thoughts go for you and your family during these difficult times. Be confident you are in good hands. In these times, family and friends are the game-changer. Just cooperate, have faith and trust in your medical team. All is going to be alright. Our prayers are with you and your family; they will comfort you at 8 a.m. "Eye of the tiger, boss! See you in a few weeks." – Carlos (Mexico)

"My wife and I are praying for you – I know you are as tough as nails." – Koush (Canada)

"Your positivity and good humor in what must be a worrying time is a testament to you as a man and as a leader." – Juan (United Kingdom)

"You make a difference. You have the love and respect of those around you. When I say take the necessary time to get better, I mean it. We all mean it. Collectively, we are here for you. We will continue to be here for you. You surrounded yourself with those who believe in you. That's why you know in your heart you can count on every one of us to keep things going while you recover." – Randy (Florida)

"Hey, chief, be patient. Be strong, don't forget that our Dear Lord is always testing us, as your most enthusiastic student I have much to learn from you, we must keep walking. Every Tuesday and Sunday my wife and I go to the church, we are Catholic. Yesterday all our prayers were for you. I hope the best, and you are the best. Don't forget it." – Javier (Columbia)

I will always cherish these notes. Their demonstration of compassion and caring is a generous gift for my soul. The lesson is that it is okay to confide in others, even in the darkest hours of your life. When I experience this overwhelming kindness from others, I make a mental note to myself that one day I, too, can be as helpful to someone in their time of need.

Chapter 1:

My wife's intimate plea

The magnitude of emotions and thoughts is overwhelming. Here I am, coming to realize I have crippled my wife, not knowing how she will cope without me if I do not survive. Although I have invested heavily in my career to provide for her, I feel like I failed at preparing her to live alone. And I still have questions. Have I honestly come to terms with my mortality? Where is the manual that explains how to do this? Have I played catch with my son for the last time? Have I made love with my wife for the last time? These are just a few of the questions I ask myself as the clock ticks on.

It is Sunday—the day before surgery. June and I decide to eat lunch at the place we go to every Sunday: Pappadeaux Seafood

Kitchen. Rarely do we have a server other than Francis. Today is no exception. We are such creatures of habit that we do not look at the menu, and we don't order. Francis knows what we like. The moment he sees us, he greets us, always with a smile, checks to see if we want the usual, and then proceeds to delight us with a wonderful meal and excellent service intermixed with friendly conversation. He is such a lovely, welcoming, and accommodating person. Today, our interaction with Francis centers around what will take place the following morning.

That week is Mardi Gras week at the restaurant; the wait staff is all wearing company-issued bright, colorful shirts for the occasion. After lunch, Francis surprises us both by picking up the tab and giving me a brand new Pappadeaux Mardi Gras shirt, including instructions telling me I need to survive the surgery so I can come back next year and get another shirt. It is so generous of him and the Pappadeaux restaurant.

Ice storms are predicted to be moving into Dallas at approximately 5:30 p.m. that evening. Outside, it is bitter cold, the wind is howling, and the sky is a sea of gray clouds, offering no hint of sunlight as far as we can see. Ice storms create dangerous driving conditions. They generally start with heavy rain—no snow—followed by a deep freeze. In a matter of two hours, the roads can be completely iced over. Driving a car in an ice storm is like driving on an ice skating rink. There is no snow to provide support and the average motorist in Texas does not usually have special tires for winter driving. When the ice storms hit, pretty much everything shuts down: transportation, schools, and businesses.

We are due to check in at the hospital at 5:30 a.m. the next day. Not knowing how adverse the road conditions will be, we decide to leave our home for the evening and check in to a hotel that is literally across the street from the hospital, a one-minute walk away. Although I want to be in the comfort of my home with my wife and familiar surroundings, I think it is best if we go to the hotel and relieve ourselves of the anxiety from having to drive fifteen miles on the ice at 4:30 a.m. to make a 5:30 check-in time.

As we walk from the parking lot into the hotel, I look at the heart hospital across the street, wondering where in the facility I will be and if that is where my life will cease. I keep these thoughts to myself, not wanting to alarm June any further. After checking in to the hotel and getting to the room, I lie down on the bed and turn on the television. June begins her usual routine of unpacking and organizing. Unlike me, she needs a set of clothes for the day of surgery and a change of clothes for the following morning since she plans to spend the night in the hospital room with me. We agree to keep the hotel room an extra night so that June can have a place to shower, change clothes, or take a break as she needs to.

June approaches the bed, sits down, and says, "Kevin, there is something I would like to ask of you."

"Of course," I reply as I turn the television off, wondering what she could possibly want to ask. Little did I know that we were about to have a moment of deep, intimate, real communication like never before in our marriage.

At this moment, the only sound is the humming of the heater pumping warm air into the room. June takes my hand and begins by telling me she realizes that what she is about to ask is selfish. She looks down, almost ashamed of what she wants to ask. She continues, "Often, with this type of surgery, patients have later reported seeing the light, a light that draws them to it. If you see this light, you may see loved ones that have passed, like your parents. You will be tempted to enter the light and be with them. As selfish as this is, I am asking you to resist the light. Please don't go; do not give in."

All I think is that her fear is far greater than I suspected. To comfort her as best I can, I make light of the situation, telling her that if I see the light and my parents, I will resist it by waving at them and saying that I can't come now, but I will see them later.

Not surprisingly, there was not a hint of comfort in June's eyes as I try to keep the discussion light. I try to console her by saying everything is going to be okay and that I will resist the light and wake up to see her after the surgery. She then says to me, "There is something else you should know." She explains that another thing that happens often with this type of surgery is patients report floating in the operating room, hovering over the operation that is taking place. She tells me not to be afraid if I experience it. She suggests I embrace it while working to come back into my body. Admittedly, this frightens me.

All I can say is: "Yes, of course; I will do that."

We lie down together, holding hands, pretending to watch television, grasping for any sense of normalcy we can find in the moment.

Oddly, after lying together for a couple of hours, June caressing my arm, I begin to feel less anxious. With each passing minute, I feel a change come over me, a calming, a sort of peace. I do not want June to be left without a husband and Kevin Jr. without a father. Believing this is God's way of preparing me, I pray, "God, I am so worried about June and Kevin Jr. Please comfort them in ways only you can do. If it is your will that my time on this earth is over, then please take me. I faithfully surrender to you and your wishes."

At that precise moment, I come to terms with my mortality. The next thing I remember is the alarm going off at 3:30 a.m. June gets up to shower, and I think, "It's game time."

Chapter 8

Game time – Bucket list and prayer

lthough the hospital is just across the parking lot from the hotel, we decide to drive the very short distance to the hospital entrance rather than risk slipping on the ice and injuring ourselves. Walking into the hospital so early on this bitterly cold morning is a haunting experience. There is no one in the lobby besides June and me. We arrive at the admissions area and take a seat. Checking into the hospital is a familiar process since I was recently there for the cardiac catheterization procedure.

After completing the paperwork, the admitting clerk escorts us to an area in the hospital that contains several beds, each of which has privacy curtains. Here is where I will change into my gown and have the IV started while they prepare the operating room. I have to remove my wedding band and contact lens, making it difficult for me to see more than five to seven feet away. I wonder if this is the last time I will see the ring on my finger. It is cold in this area of the hospital because of the frigid and icy conditions outside.

My son, Kevin, is with us. It is a somewhat awkward time... neither of us knows what to talk about, so we make small talk. I can sense my son is frightened; he has never seen his dad in this situation. Growing up, he looked up to me as a robust and indestructible man, a provider and protector. This morning he sees me getting ready to fight for my life and at the mercy of the surgical team. I tell him I will see him in a few hours and not to worry about a thing.

Even though she does not say it, June is scared. As a registered nurse, she is wearing what I call her "game face." But, as her husband, I can see past the emotional disguise she is wearing. She, too, doesn't know if she will see me alive again once I am wheeled away to surgery. It is a surreal situation to be in the presence of family fully aware that this may be the last smile, the last hug, the final touch.

A nurse comes in to start my IV. After a few minutes of looking for a vein, and one failed attempt at getting it started, she says she will have the anesthesiologist start the IV once I am in the operating room. She places a large, warm blanket over me. This all-encompassing heat penetrating my body, warming me up, is quite soothing and comforting. My mind wanders. There must be someone in this hospital who washes, folds, and organizes these blankets for patients. This person probably does not know what an excellent service they provide, and, most likely, they never come in contact with patients. I think, "Someday, I would like to meet this person and express my thanks and appreciation for the role they play in helping patients by making these blankets available."

Dr. Moore comes in, looking relaxed and calm with a hint of focus and purpose. I expect to see him dressed in a white lab coat, but this morning he is wearing jeans and a sweatshirt. "What a cool guy," I think. He smiles as he greets June and Kevin Jr. He then asks me, "Are you ready?"

I reply, "Did you bring your A game?"

"Yes, I did."

"Then I am ready. Let's do this."

He asks me if I need anything, then tells me he will see me shortly before leaving to change and prepare for the operation.

Even though I appear calm and ready, there are a million questions seeping into my mind as I lie there with Kevin on one side of the bed and June on the other.

"Have I played catch with my son for the last time?"

"Have I danced with my wife for the last time?"

"Will I never make love with my wife again?"

"Will my unborn grandchild ever meet their grandpa?"

"I can die at any moment. Will it hurt? How long might I suffer?"

"As I head to surgery, will this be my last hug and kiss with my wife and family?"

"Have I come to peace with my Maker correctly? What is the correct way to do it?"

"How is my wife going to cope if I don't come through this?"

I see a man approaching me. Without my contact lens, I am unable to make out who he is. As he arrives at my bedside, I notice he is holding a crucifix.

"Hello, Kevin. My name is Rob. I am the hospital chaplain."

I am surprised that a chaplain came to see me. It is somewhat frightening. I realize that this is it; it's time. Chaplain Rob asks if I have religion in my life. I tell him I believe in Jesus Christ as my savior. He asks if it would be okay for him to say a prayer. I tell him, "Of course." He proceeds to pray, starting with thanking the Lord for our daily blessing of life. He then asks God to watch over me during the surgery and to guide the surgeon and his team to perform to the best of their abilities. I thank him for the visit and the prayer. I hope June and Kevin are not frightened because of the chaplain's unexpected visit.

It's never too late for prayer; God will forgive you of all sin; all you need to do is to invite the Lord into your heart as your Savior.

A hospital worker comes over, saying they are ready for me now. She prepares the bed so that she can transport me to the operating room. I give Kevin and June a hug. I kiss June, telling her that I love her and I will see her soon. Just before we exit the area, I turn and give June and Kevin a smile and wave. And as I am wheeled through the door and into the hallway that leads to the operating room, I feel a profound sense that I am being prayed over. I wonder if I am feeling the prayers of my colleagues at the same time. It feels prayers are pouring over me as we progress down the hallway. I am feeling the power of prayer like never before. I immerse myself in the thought of others praying for me all at the same time and how nice that is. I decide to say a prayer myself.

"Dear God,

I have come to terms with my mortality; my precious wife is not prepared for my passing. I believe in you as my Savior, and I am sorry for the sinning I have done in my life, I ask for your forgiveness. Please take me today if it is your will to do so. If my life is to be spared, I pray that you will allow me to complete a bucket list I have created for myself. These are the most important things I want to achieve during my remaining years.

#1 Dance with my wife again
#2 Hold hands with my wife and take a walk
#3 Meet my unborn grandchild

Thank you for the life I have lived thus far. I give myself and my fate entirely up to you."

The doors swing open as I enter the operating room. I see lots of people moving around, doing whatever they do to prepare for this surgery. As they wheel me around, lining me up next to the surgical table, I spot the heart-lung machine and a gentleman working with it. I think, as I am looking at him, the perfusionist, "He is the person who will be keeping me alive during the surgery." It is quite sobering to see the actual equipment that is going to keep me alive, as well as the man who will operate and monitor that equipment during the surgery.

A man introduces himself as the physician who will harvest the vein from my left leg to use as one of the bypasses. The anesthesiologist sits at my side and begins the IV that could not be started earlier. He explains that he will be the one keeping a close eye on my vitals, my sleep, and where I need to be during the surgery. He says that once they put me under, they will insert a breathing tube (endotracheal tube). It is a flexible plastic tube that is placed in the trachea, or windpipe, through the mouth or nose to help the patient breathe. He says he will also be inserting various ports so he can inject medicine at a moment's notice if needed.

The nurse who will be with me during the surgery—and who will provide updates to June—also introduces herself.

The room is far more high-tech than I imagined, with many monitors and various pieces of equipment surrounding me. I also did not realize until then how many people are in the operating room during open-heart surgery.

The anesthesiologist tells me I am going to feel some medicine flow into the vein, which will relax me. I do not remember feeling relaxed, or anything at all, after he speaks to me.

Below is the timeline for the surgery.

9:11 a.m.	Surgery begins
10:40 a.m.	Placed on heart-lung machine
12:25 p.m.	Third bypass started
1:40 p.m.	Surgery finishes
4:00 p.m.	Got to see June

I hear a man's voice speaking to me, "Kevin, it's okay, just relax, just relax."

I sense something being pulled out of my throat. I have a brief choking sensation followed by the sense that everything is okay. My head is foggy, making it challenging to comprehend what is going on, but I later realize that sensation is coming from the removal of the endotracheal tube. I must have fallen back to sleep because the next thing I remember is being in my hospital room: room 610.

Chapter 9:

Room 610 – Hospital of Angels

*J*genuinely believe all big things are made possible through little things—little things that leave lasting impressions. Something big is about to happen in room 610 at the heart hospital.

That something is Life 2.0.

In the operating room at a hospital, our surgeons hold our hearts in their hands and restart them. In the operating room of life, our caregivers hold our lives in their hearts and restart, reshape, and mold them in ways we do not imagine possible, a way I call Life 2.0. As patients, we move on, we move forward, but we never forget.

You are never left behind.

Day 1 (surgery)

I am interrupted by the familiar sensation of waking up; however, I feel as though an oppressive fog surrounds me. It obscures my vision and hinders my breathing. I do not know where I am, and it is eerily quiet. My brain has trouble processing what is happening. I feel blinded by the sudden sensory overload and lost in a hazy version of my reality, causing me to desperately want to get a grip on my surroundings.

Opening my eyes for the first time, as I lie in the hospital room having just had open-heart surgery, I am greeted by the familiar smile, loving words, and gentle touch of my beloved wife. Even in my fog, I feel relieved to be alive.

But I see fear and despair in her eyes…. I remain quiet as I gaze back at her.

The fog begins to lift, and my vision begins to clear. I realize I am attached to machines by long strings of wire; these machines are beeping and making sputtering noises. I have IVs in my arms, chest, and neck. My chest is wrapped in thick bandaging. I wonder, "Am I okay?"

My thoughts are interrupted by: "Hello Kevin. My name is Brandon, and I will be your nurse today. You are out of surgery. You are in cardiac ICU, and you are okay. You are doing just fine." He says all this with a warm and comforting smile. In just a matter of minutes, I observe that Brandon is confident, experienced, knowledgeable, compassionate, and passionate about being an exceptional nurse. I sense he is very good at his job. He also has a good sense of humor to compliment his "take charge" demeanor. Even though I just came from major surgery, I feel safe in his care. I am glad he is with me.

I know that June, having practiced as a registered nurse for many years, is observing how well he cares for me. She knows what good healthcare looks like. She will be watching over me like a hawk. Brandon steps just outside the door to attend to something at the nurse's station. June comes to my side and tells me she is very impressed with the medical team that is caring for me; she says they are good. June tells me Brandon is an excellent nurse. I quickly feel at ease just knowing she is confident in those who are caring for me. I think I am lucky, but I am about to learn that the entire nursing organization is world-class.

I wake up again, realizing I fell back asleep. June is still at my side. I apologize for going to sleep on her. She smiles, saying, "You are tired. You need to rest. Don't worry; I will be here."

As we converse, I take inventory of what is hooked up to me. First, I notice three tubes coming out of my abdominal area, approximately five inches directly above my naval. Brandon confirms my suspicion that these are drainage tubes. I then discover metal wires are coming out of my upper abdomen area, just below my sternum. Brandon explains that these wires are leads that are attached to my heart in case they need to pace my heart for any reason.

Surprisingly, I don't have any pain, although I soon find out that this pain-free surgery is temporary. The pain in my chest is mounting. Brandon administers a dose of morphine and tells me to let them know when I am in pain. He wants to stay ahead of it and keep me comfortable.

When Brandon steps out of the room, June asks me if I remember seeing the light and if by chance I was out of body watching over the procedure. I tell her there was no light, no hovering, nothing. I can tell she is relieved.

I wake up again—again not realizing I had fallen asleep—to Dr. Moore entering my room. He greets us and tells me the surgery went well and explains that I had three bypasses, called grafts, put in. The report from Dr. Moore was excellent; he was able to use both internal mammary arteries and the one vein harvested from my leg for the grafts. He sits down and begins to explain the next steps of the plan. I will have a respiratory specialist come by each day to oversee breathing exercises. Dr. Moore explains that they want to get my lungs back to full capacity as soon as possible. I will also have to get on my feet soon and start to walk. I look at him with a funny expression, as if to say, "There is no way I am going to get on my feet and start walking." He asks me a few more questions and charts my responses. About the time it appears, his visit is over, I say, "Dr. Moore, I have a question for you."

"Sure, anything you would like to ask," he replies.

"Did you have a hard time restarting my heart?"

It was as if he had seen a ghost. He looks right at me, pauses for what seems like an eternity, and says, "A little. I had to shock it a few extra times to get it going."

"Thank you, I was just curious," I say.

Once Dr. Moore leaves the room, June asks why I asked him that question.

"I heard them, June. I heard him talking. Although I am not entirely sure, it sounded like, 'C'mon Kevin.' I did not see the light. I did not float in the operating room. But I did hear Dr. Moore's voice. I sense it was during the time he was restarting my heart," I explain.

"Okay, time to get up and walk," Brandon says. I am petrified. I feel weak and unstable. Brandon shows me how I will hug a pillow and position myself to get up without putting pressure on the incision in my chest, avoiding pain as much as possible. Once I am sitting upright on the bed, he puts a support strap on me, which is used to prevent me from falling when they are assisting me with walking.

Up we go. I am on my feet with Brandon and a nurse's aide helping me. I feel as though I am going to pass out, not even sure if I can take a step. But Brandon tells me I can do it, so off I go on my first walk after surgery. I do not get very far, maybe twenty or thirty feet from the room. That is all I can do before I am ready to get back into bed. Brandon explains that, over the next few days, I need to be able to walk the perimeter of the ICU area, around the nurse's station, and back to my room. That objective seems insurmountable. But because Brandon is so helpful and encouraging, I want to show him I can do this; I want to exceed his expectations. He tells me that walking and getting my lungs back to normal is the best way to get myself discharged; it's my ticket out.

Around 6 p.m., Brandon briefs the night nurses on my condition and prepares them before his shift ends. Brandon is an upstanding person, so encouraging to me. He loves his profession; perhaps that is why he is so good at it. He tells June and me goodnight as he heads out. June is going to spend the night in the room with me.

Other than being woken up every hour to test my blood sugar, I anticipate getting through the night okay. However, around 10 p.m., I wake to the machines making all kinds of noises. It's as if something is happening…. June is awake. The nurse comes in the room and stares at the equipment, saying nothing. He leaves, but moments later, he and three others are in my room. Something is happening; I ask what is going on. My heart rate and blood pressure are dropping, and my electrolyte levels are not normal. I can see June is frightened. For all I know, I am going into cardiac arrest. One of the people in the room hooks my metal wires up to something and tells me they are going to try and pace my heart, which essentially means establishing a regular rhythm. While this is happening, they inject something into my IV, stating that it should help.

In about fifteen minutes, I can tell they are relieved. Whatever was going on with me is now okay. Neither June nor I can sleep the rest of the night; it was quite a miserable experience. They continue to test my blood sugars hourly, and the respiratory therapist has me do my exercises a couple of times during the night. I wasn't a fan of those exercises because inhaling from the device the respiratory therapist brought along was very painful around the incision on my chest.

Day 2

It's 7 a.m. Brandon is back.

June tells him how happy she is to see him and explains that she does not have the same level of confidence in the night nurse as she does him. Brandon is humble, and he thanks June for the compliment. June soon heads back to the hotel to shower and get some rest.

Lifting the phone to order breakfast causes a flare-up of pain. They now have me on a regular pain medication regimen, so I look forward to the next dose. As I wait for breakfast, a gentle giant of a man enters my room. With a reassuring and comforting smile, he tells me he is here to clean my room, does want to disturb me, and would be happy to come back if now is not convenient.

I tell him, "By all means, sir, come on in. Now is a good time."

As I watch him sweep, empty the trash, and clean up, I notice he appears to take great pride in his work. I can tell he is happy with the way he applies himself to his work and does so with a smile. "What a ray of sunshine this gentleman is," I think to myself as I ask him his name.

"Alvin," he says, pausing for a moment to send a smile my way.

He wishes me a good day and once again apologizes for disturbing my rest. As he leaves, I am left with an impression of this good man that will stay with me for a long time. I think about how I hope I can see him again one day.

Little do I know that Alvin will play an extraordinarily significant role in my future.

A while later, June comes back. She is happy to see me and is looking refreshed. I do not comment, but I know she is still fatigued. She tells me how impressed she is with everyone's kindness. In particular, the valet attendant provides some comforting words to June as she returns to the hospital. He tells her, "I know your husband is going to be okay and will be able to go home soon. If there is anything I can do so that your time here is as pleasant as possible, please let me know."

I have been feeling helpless to minister to my wife and comfort her. I am so impressed and happy that others are helping her cope by kindly offering their compassion, understanding, and rays of hope. My experience with valet attendants is that they want to park the car so they can later return it and collect a tip. It's just a job. I am duly impressed with this gentleman who is so kind to my wife in her time of need. I make a note that his ministry to her is also a ministry to me. He probably doesn't know that his small and straightforward act of kindness and compassion makes its way into room 610 and warms my heart.

Terri, a nurse practitioner specialist, comes to visit. Her upbeat and bubbly personality quickly catches my attention. She explains that her role is to be Dr. Moore's eyes and ears when he is not in the hospital. She tells me that everything looks good and is progressing the way it should. I confide in Terri that the pain is approaching unbearable. She tells me that much of the pain and discomfort stem from the drainage tubes. Once those are out, I should feel much better. Unfortunately, those won't come out for another day or two. The entire time Terri is with me, I am not as consumed with my pain. She is such a bubbly person; it lifts my spirits to be around her. She is a personable and gifted person who makes me feel as though I am the only patient in the hospital.

I look forward to seeing her again.

My breathing exercises, monitored by the respiratory specialist, continue. I still don't like doing them. However, I do realize that one of the essential items for recovery and getting out of the hospital is having my lung capacity in the normal range. I have to accept the pain and power through it.

Two ladies come into my room, carrying one of the walking straps. I assume this means I have to absorb more pain by sitting up in bed in preparation for a walk. They introduce themselves. Lydia, one of the rehabilitation specialists, is very patient with me and impresses me with her encouragement and focused attention. Once they get me on my feet, I turn to Lydia and give her a look of uncertainty. I'm wondering if she can hold me up all by herself if I fall. Lydia appears to be a very fit lady, but I am a large man. As we exit my room and turn to walk down the hall, she says, "Is my husband talking good care of you?"

Oh my goodness, she is Brandon's wife! How surprised and delighted I am to learn of this. I give her an earful about how magnificent Brandon is. At one point, I see him at the nurse's station.

"Hey Brandon," I say with a hint of arrogance and humor. "I am going to take your wife for a walk. When do I need to have her back?" We all have a good laugh and off I go on my walk. Approaching the halfway mark, I get incredibly nauseous. I am dizzy, feeling like I am going to faint. Lydia has me stop and be still until I can get control of my senses and feel stable enough to continue. Walking back to the room takes a very long time. All I want to do is lie in bed and close my eyes.

Brandon comes into the room with Editha, a nurse who will be taking care of me in the evening. She has short, dark hair and a calming and comforting presence about her. Editha immediately impresses me as a sweet, caring, and compassionate person. She has an extraordinary impact on my recovery and outlook on life, even though I do not know this at the time. They leave the room so that Brandon can update her on my condition and make arrangements for a shift change.

It is getting late in the day; I see that June needs a break. I encourage June to spend the night at home instead of another restless night in the hospital room. Reluctantly, she agrees. I give her a hug and a kiss, assuring her I will be fine and that I look forward to seeing her tomorrow. She does not admit it, but I can tell by the look in her eye that she is uncomfortable leaving after what happened the night before when the machines were alarming.

As June leaves the room, I can see the staff at the nursing station give her smiles and kind words. I am comforted seeing others minister to her. I know she is feeling lonely and frightened. Just as I see her disappear around the corner toward the elevator, I notice the room is abnormally quiet. I very apparently feel alone. The silence invites reflection. What led me here? What path do I take moving forward?

Emotionally, I feel as though I am a failure, letting my family and work colleagues down by getting sick at such an early age. Feelings of depression and anger evaporate any remaining positive motivation I have. I eventually relegate myself to sleep in order to bypass the depression and physical pain I feel, no pun intended. Sleep will numb me. It will be my escape from the predicament I find myself in.

Although everyone tells me the surgery is a success, it is hard for me to believe this wholeheartedly and be confident that I am okay. After all, I had no symptoms before or after surgery, yet I was on the verge of a fatal cardiac event. How could I be sure that, in the absence of symptoms, even after surgery, I was okay?

I couldn't.

I am woken by Editha telling me she needs to bathe me, administer some pain medications, and test my blood sugar levels. The blood sugar test involves drawing a tiny amount of blood from my fingertip so the machine can report my blood sugar levels. I am confident I will not be getting much sleep this night with the blood sugar test every hour.

Throughout the evening, Editha continues to check on me often. From time to time, I see her looking at me through the glass window, which the nurses use to keep an eye on their patients while they are not in the room. Everything about her is pleasant. She makes me feel comfortable when we speak with one another. Editha is very knowledgeable; she can answer every question I ask regarding my condition and recovery. I get the impression she loves her career. I am fascinated by her passion for giving expert care. After all, she works all night and then has a husband and children to care for when she is off work. Her stamina, passion, and care can only come from her love of nursing and helping others.

I talk to her about my pain. She tells me I will feel much better once the drainage tubes are removed and she will stay on top of administering pain medications so I can get by until that happens. The next time she tests my blood sugar, she asks me to guess what the result will be. I tell her what I think then ask her to also take a guess. Being a competitive person, I do not like to lose, but in this case, I did lose and was completely happy to do so. This game of guessing blood sugar goes on all night as each hour comes around. Overall, Editha was right more often than I was. After a few times, I begin to look forward to each successive test.

One time I pretend to be asleep as she enters my room. She wipes my finger with alcohol, something she always does before drawing blood. I open my eyes, smile at her, and guess the result. She is tickled once she realizes I am not asleep and wanted to surprise her.

Before I sleep, I think about how kind Editha is to me. I am grateful to have an opportunity to meet her and get to know her, even though the circumstances are not ideal…or are they? I think of the genuine, caring, and compassionate people we have come in contact with from the moment I was admitted to the hospital. They are all around me. They all work hard to help me and guide me through this phase of recovery. They do so because they care, not because it is a job.

Perhaps I shouldn't worry so much about myself and my selfish needs but, instead, absorb the notion that others are putting their life on hold to care for me. They put my life ahead of their own. Perhaps there is something to learn from what I am experiencing.

Day 3

This morning I meet Beth; she will be my nurse today. Brandon is very good with patients who have just come out of surgery. In contrast, I will later observe that Beth is very good at helping patients become self-sufficient by working diligently with them on breathing exercises, walking, and preparing to leave the hospital. At first, I am not sure I will like this. Whereas Brandon and Editha do everything for me, Beth wants to see me get up and use the bathroom or take a walk unattended. I notice that Beth is not in my room as often as the others were. I soon realize this is how it must be, how I must transition from being catered to every moment to becoming an independent self-starter in my recovery. I discover this as Beth encourages me when I pass a milestone in my recovery; this motivates me.

For the first time, I have a desire to give back to the employees of the hospital. I want to demonstrate to them that their efforts and sacrifices are not in vain but that they make a difference to the patients and impact their lives in the most profound and positive ways.

I want them all to be proud of me and to genuinely feel how much of a difference they make in the lives of their patients and their patients' families. Motivated to put forth the effort and work hard, I decide to attempt getting to my feet without anyone's help. As I lie in bed, strategizing how I am going to pull this off, I mentally rehearse the steps I was taught for how to do this. I eventually find myself sitting up in bed—what an achievement. I must have done something wrong because the pain is mounting in my chest. I don't think I can stand up; I also don't think I can lie down. I am stuck, unable to move forward or return to my former position.

I see a lady busily and briskly pass my room. A second later, she backs up and from the door asks, "Hi there, could you use some help?"

I must look desperate.

I explain that I am in pain and I am not able to move from this position. With a look of empathy, she enters my room and very patiently helps me back into bed without any increase in my pain levels. I thank her for helping me and tell her how kind it was for her to do so. She smiles and says that is why she works here: to help people. She then introduces herself; her name is Carla. After she leaves, I note how I met yet another person who loves to help others, who puts their own needs to the side. When she first walked past my room, I could tell she is a very busy person, but she stopped to attend to me, a stranger. A little while later, Beth comes into the room, and, with a smile, says, "I hear ya tried to get up and walk on your own."

Explaining my embarrassment for failing, I ask how she knew what I attempted. She replied, "Our head of cardiac ICU nursing told me. She is the one who helped you."

I am even more impressed that someone looking after a team of nurses caring for cardiac ICU patients took time out of their day to help me. She could have called someone to help, but she didn't. She wanted to help me at that moment. My experience with Carla and her spontaneous act of kindness makes another lasting impression.

The nurse practitioner, Terri, visits me. Good news, she is going to remove two of the three drainage tubes. Removing them is supposed to make me feel better. However, I have some apprehension; I have never had tubes pulled out of my body. Terri explains it does not necessarily hurt, but it feels strange.

Okay, here we go.

On my third breath, I exhale and close my eyes. The sensation of having a tube pulled from my body is something I have never experienced. After a few seconds, I am relieved to know there is one down and one to go.

"All done," she says.

"Terri, I thought you were going to remove two of them."

She smiles like the cat that ate the canary and says, "I took two out at the same time."

That is awesome. She checks my wires, bandages, and IVs and lets me know she will most likely remove the third tube tomorrow. Just like all others, Terri demonstrates that her priority is patient comfort and well-being during recovery by sparing me the anxiety and sensation of removing the drainage tubes separately. This little act of kindness makes a lasting impression, signifying that we sometimes have the opportunity to double the impact of our goodness toward others.

That evening, after June leaves to go home, a male nurse enters my room to check on me. He introduces himself as Roy and lets me know he is helping Beth out and doing patient rounds. Once he determines I am stable and comfortable, I explain my difficulty completing the breathing exercises because of the pain I feel in my chest. He reminds me of the two most important tasks to conquer before Dr. Moore releases me: 1) get my lungs to a healthy state and 2) demonstrate I can walk the designated path. He provides some tips on how to master the breathing exercise and also helps with my techniques to get on my feet and back to the bed. He spends a fair amount of time with me. I wonder why a nurse not assigned to me would take this amount of time to help me progress. I am impressed by his generosity and genuine interest in helping me. That day, Roy makes a lasting impression on me; I can learn from him too.

As Editha begins her shift, I look forward to playing our blood sugar guessing game. Tonight is going to be different. I have enjoyed her sense of humor, so it is time for me to play a joke on her. She is accustomed to seeing me as she looks through the observation window or when she enters the room. The trick I want to play is to leave the room when she is not looking. The time comes as she finishes checking in on me. Just after she goes, I work to sit up so that I can get on my feet and hide. I am in more pain for some reason, but manage to sit on the edge of the bed with my feet planted on the floor. I begin the move to stand up, and the pain is too much for me to finish. I stop, realizing I have made a mistake by not using the pillow I am supposed to use when getting up or lying down. Eventually, I manage to lie back down, my chest throbbing with pain. When Editha comes back, I ask her to administer some pain medication, letting her know my pain level is high. She gives me a look of confusion as she tries to figure out why I am in such pain. Little does she know it is because of a practical joke I tried to play on her, which backfired.

I don't tell her what I was doing until many months later, but she is rather amused when I do.

We settle into our routine for the evening. After a couple of rounds of the blood sugar guessing game, she lets me know she is not working the next day and will not be with me during the night. This news saddens me. After all, she is a godsend.

It is not until long after my discharge from the hospital that I realize what Editha is doing by playing the blood sugar guessing game. She is using it to distract my mind from the pain. Having me play this game is a little thing, but one that creates a lifelong impression, simply because of her unselfish pursuit to give the very best possible cardiac care to her patients. My experiences with Editha eventually serve as a key in my awakening to Life 2.0.

I often refer to Editha as the modern-day of Florence Nightingale. Florence Nightingale is arguably the most famous nurse in the history of medical care. She fundamentally changed the role of nursing in hospitals and was a key figure in introducing new professional training standards. She also established a training school for nurses in London.

Editha and Florence both possess the pure love of caring for others—not because it is their job to do so, but because it is who they are.

I am now inspired to be an expert patient, wanting to show them they make a difference.

Day 4

Today is the first day I complete the entire walk that I must complete for them to considering releasing me. As I return to from this inaugural walk, I see Beth standing just outside of my door. I let her know I made it around the entire floor. The smile she gives is as impressive as the northern lights.

Loudly, she claps her hands, and while gesturing me to high five, she says, "Yes! You are my rock star, Kevin. I knew you could do it. Way to go!"

I am happy to achieve this walk but feel a rush of exhilaration knowing my primary caregivers provided the nourishment I needed with their acknowledgment and encouragement.

I am valued; I am relevant; I am important.

There is power in the little things others do, particularly when they ask for nothing in return.

Of the many things Beth could have said to me, she could not have picked a more powerful one than: "You are my rock star." Little does Beth know that is what my work colleagues call me, and, most of all, it makes me feel like I am progressing. I am reminded to never underestimate the powerful impact of words.

Today has been a good day. Beth makes me feel good about myself. Terri, the nurse practitioner, pays me a visit to remove the third drainage tube and the three wires inserted into my heart. Once the third tube is removed, I immediately feel relief from pain in my chest and pressure on my lungs. Removing the three wires is another a strange sensation. She has me perform similar breathing techniques for the removal of the wires as she did when removing the tubes. She then tugs lightly on the wire, breaking it loose from the heart muscle, then pulls it out. During the extraction of the wire, I do feel a slight burning sensation in the skin surrounding the metal wire. The first two are easy. Then she goes for the third, and, as she tugs, it won't come out. It's stuck!

"What now?" I think to myself. "This is making me very anxious; it is not supposed to happen this way."

Terri smiles and says, "Let's try it again." This time she wiggles the wire slightly, and it comes right out. I am so relieved.

Day 5 (discharge)

Terri stops by to see me once again with her bubbly, energetic, and comforting personality. She informs me that I am progressing well enough for her to seek Dr. Moore's approval for me to be released today, adding that it is up to me if I want that. It catches me off guard to be allowed to make the decision based solely on how I feel. Giving me her support and the choice of leaving or staying another night is another selfless act by a member of this healthcare organization. I decide to go home today; I miss my home. I miss my bed, and, most of all, I miss sleeping with my wife.

Terri will call Dr. Moore, get his approval, and then have the discharge paperwork put in motion. Before she leaves the room, she says, "Kevin, please call me any time if you need anything or wish to ask questions. No question is too silly or trivial." A hug follows her encouragement. She is a remarkable and special lady.

A member of the cardiac rehabilitation team visits to explain the rehabilitation program I will follow and the locations in the city where I can attend. My program will begin four weeks after surgery with sessions three times per week for twelve weeks. Even though there are rehabilitation locations closer to my home, I decide I want to participate in the program at the hospital.

As I wait for the discharge paperwork to be completed, I reflect on my experiences with the people we have come in contact with at the hospital.

There is a sense of community and teamwork throughout the entire hospital. The approach seems to be to treat guests and their families with dignity and respect while working extremely hard to save and extend life. This approach is not what I usually perceive modern-day healthcare's to be.

Employees, regardless of job function, are happy to be there. Each one exhibits pride in their contributions. They are delighted to be there, dedicated and passionate about the patients, their families, and their loved ones. The guests are made to feel relevant and valuable.

The sum of the parts, the little things that make lasting impressions, represent something far more significant than I have ever experienced.

Unparalleled exemplary care throughout the entire organization sets the stage for something big coming in my life. These special people will forever be etched into my feelings of eternal gratitude, primarily because of the little things they do.

As I contemplate my experience, I realize what this organization was doing for me. Their knowledge, skill, and teamwork give me confidence. Their encouragement gives me hope. Their attitude and approach give me a life to live.

Compassion, smiles, pride, passion, protection, and making sure the guests know they are relevant sparks an "I'm okay, I can do this" attitude as I move forward.

It occurs to me that one person or function did not predominantly provide the little things; they came from exceptional people, regardless of their role. Personnel who do not come in direct contact with patients also make lasting impressions, and most do not imagine that to be possible. Perhaps they do something for a family member, which provides comfort and peace for the patient. Maybe they do something for a colleague who comes in contact with a patient and the goodness is passed on to the patient. One never knows the power and depth of little things. The valet attendants, the people who clean and fold surgical blankets, and the people who clean rooms are exceptional. Everyone makes an impact on the life of a patient, their family, and their loved ones with the little things they do every day.

Throughout my stay in the hospital, I am witness to an over-abundance of little things that make lasting impressions and fuel my recognition of the good in humanity. I wonder if I have never opened my eyes…for now, I can see.

I see tenderness, compassion, protection, safety, kindness, humor, smiles, unrelenting care, gentleness, sincerity, and humble-ness in people all around me. It is how I imagine Angels to be. I was in room 610 in a hospital of Angels. I indeed met many Angels during my stay; they walk among us.

"Time to go," a nurse's aide says as she enters the room with a wheelchair. She asks June to get the car and pull up outside, and she will bring me down.

Beth hugs me and says, "Take care, rock star. Come back and visit."

I decide that one day I will indeed come back and visit. Perhaps it will be my turn to give back.

Between my room and the elevator is the nurse's station. As I am wheeled to the elevator, passing by the nurse's station, I raise my right hand as high as I can, saying, "Thank you for saving my life, I will not forget you."

Smile after smile breaks out across the team of nurses present. At that precise moment, something catches my eye in my periph-eral vision. I turn my head as far to the left as I can and catch a glimpse of a nurse walking the opposite direction. Just as she is about to disappear from sight, she turns, looking over her left shoulder at me. What I see in her eyes, for that split second, I have never seen before in my life. It is spiritual.

The entire trip home, June and I discuss my care and how we will cope without having the help from the hospital. I think June is very nervous and thinks that she needs to be on high alert. I try to comfort her by explaining that they would not release me unless everything was fine.

That does not seem to help.

She begins to create a plan in the event of an emergency. During moments of pause in our conversation, I am still struck by what I saw as I left the hospital—so warm, so loving, so protecting. Could it be what I think it is?

Indeed, this is a hospital of Angels.

Chapter 10:

Rehab – The gang, and my new friend Dan

A culmination of events and interactions leads to a turning point in my life, somewhat analogous to turning on a light switch: a short click immediately followed by light.

Life 2.0 begins to take form.

I am no different than anyone else attending cardiac rehabilitation. I enter the program focused on me, not anyone else. In some sense, it is a selfish approach, but an understandable one.

I feel relieved to be alive, but for several weeks following surgery, I refuse to admit the levels of fear, despair, and sadness I hold inside. Coming home from the hospital, I feel as though I am a broken man, riddled with imperfection, and begin to question my longevity. I wonder if I am alone in these feelings or if everyone coming home from open-heart surgery feels the same.

The quietness of our home, the stillness of my surroundings, paves the way for many thoughts to consume me. I struggle to reconcile these thoughts. I let so many people down by getting sick at such an early age. I experience depression and anger. I am motivated only by sleep, which is quickly becoming my ticket to ignoring the world around me. Once again, I contemplate the little things the nurses, food service people, and janitorial service did for me and how others ministered to my wife in kind and compassionate ways.

In many ways, I am at war with myself, fighting to keep life from pulling me down and struggling to hold on to the gifts from others. Those gifts from others are what motivate me to fight harder.

June is hypervigilant about watching over me. Sitting in a lounge chair, alternating between sleep and watching television, I notice she checks on me frequently. When I am quiet for too long, she briskly comes to ask if I am okay, and when I make any noise, she also comes running to see if I am okay. At times I think this takes her back to her nursing days—only this time, her husband is her patient. I can't think of anyone else I would want in my corner to care for me. June is loving, selfless, knowledgeable, and shows her excellence through her service. I know she is frightened of the unknown, fearful I may experience a heart attack or stroke in our home. On several occasions, I take her hand and explain that all she can do is call 9-1-1 in the event something happens, and then I try my best to assure her I am okay.

I find it odd how sensitive my chest is to the touch. I am unable to wear a shirt because of the pain when the fabric brushes over my skin. I have never felt anything like this. The sensation is due to nerve damage from cutting open the chest cavity. My surgeon tells me it is normal and that it should completely go away in about a year. I resign myself to not wearing a shirt around the house. I am given a prescription to help alleviate my surface chest pain. After a few days on the medication, I notice my nerve sensitivity is declining. However, the side effects of the drug— in my case, extreme nausea—are so significant that I have to stop taking it. I resign myself to the unrelenting pain and find ways to manage.

The rehabilitation program requires me to attend three sessions per week for twelve weeks. The classes begin at 6:30 a.m. Cardiac rehabilitation is a coordinated exercise and education program designed to help patients improve their physical endurance and strength following a cardiac event, such as a heart attack or heart surgery.

June and I attend an orientation a week before my first class. We meet Lisa, one of the cardiac registered nurses on staff. She is easy to speak with and comforting to be around. The team is comprised of cardiac care registered nurses and exercise physiologists. Lisa explains the program and what I will be doing during my sessions. She shows me how to check in and which exercise stations I will be assigned. An EKG system will monitor me throughout the entire class. Because I am a diabetic, my blood sugar is also tested at the beginning of each class. If it is below an acceptable threshold, I will not be allowed to participate. I learn that eating something to raise my blood sugar is essential for being allowed to perform the workouts.

As we discuss the plan with Lisa, I can't help but notice the other patients in the background as they work out at their respective stations. Most appear to be much older than me, another reminder of how broken I am. Some seem to be my age, but only a few look younger. As a former athlete, exercise and the level of effort I can expect to put forth are not foreign to me, and I look forward to my first class.

As I drive to the hospital on my first day of rehabilitation, I fill with anxiety and fear, and I am unable to escape a feeling of depression. The rehabilitation room is just down the hall from the hospital emergency room. As I pass the emergency room, I spot a female sitting at a desk behind a closed glass window. I am not sure what she does; however, she appears to be related to the emergency room. She glances at me as I pass by.

The doors to the rehabilitation area are locked. Several classmates are waiting just outside the door. I must look like the new guy because several introduce themselves and welcome me. I enjoy this lovely feeling of belonging as well as the acknowledgment from others.

As part of checking in, I am asked my name and birthday. I then test my blood sugar, showing the results to a staff member to get permission to begin the class. Soon I am left standing by myself as the other class members proceed to their designated stations.

"Kevin, come with me," says Lisa. She teaches me how and where to place the EKG leads on my body so I can be monitored wirelessly. I am assigned to three stations, each lasting twenty minutes. Station one is the treadmill. Station two is weight lifting, and station three is the recumbent bicycle. Lisa remains with me the entire time, demonstrating how they want me to perform at each exercise station. During the session, I begin to feel more and more comfortable as others in the class give me nods and smiles of encouragement, as if they are telling me I am doing well. Again I notice the impact the little things have on me.

Driving home after class, I think, "It is time to start taking my health more seriously, time to take control. Earlier I made a decision to be an expert patient. Perhaps I should become an expert at taking care of myself. After all, countless others are helping me to achieve that. I should learn how to eat, how to exercise, and how to take my medications. I should take control of my life and do everything possible to guide myself down a healthy path. Each week I must take the opportunity to implement a heart-healthy change in my life."

Each day I attend the class, I walk through the emergency room entrance, passing the lady who sits at the glass-enclosed desk. She gives me the warmest, most welcoming smile anyone could anticipate. After a couple of times, she includes a friendly wave with her smile. It is between 6 a.m., and 6:30 a.m., so not only is she doing a job for the emergency room, but she also always takes time to smile and acknowledge me—a stranger to her. Her compassion for others stands out to me and serves as an example of how I want to be in my interactions with others. I find myself looking forward to seeing her before each class, to receiving her smile and returning her wave. It makes me feel good—like I am an alive and welcome member of society.

I soon realize why I look forward to attending my sessions. It is not because my doctor wants me there or because I love working out. It is because this is a place where I am inspired and motivated before, during, and after each session.

Before the session begins, my classmates congregate in the waiting area. We become acquainted, we learn about each other and our reasons for being there. We all feel a mutual bond, a connection so pure that I am still motivated and inspired by the togetherness we experience months and years down the line. During that time, we laugh, we empathize…we talk about everything! I find it interesting that we all seem to enjoy arriving early and having "our" time. When we are allowed in the rehabilitation area, we all feel so comfortable with one another. We know we are about to work together, make progress together, but, most of all, we know we are going to be with one another, and it is good.

We talk to each other as we exercise, sometimes to others who are several stations away. We laugh, and it is good. The bond among us patients is further enhanced by the cardiac rehabilitation staff's encouragement and teachings. It is nice to know someone is there for us, to make sure we do things right, to remark on progress, and to help us when something isn't right, to watch over us. It feels like everyone is there for everyone else; it is good. Where else do you get a high five for a good blood pressure—or just for being alive?

After class, a few of us talk and enjoy each other's company. What a great feeling it is to be in communion with another person with whom you share a common bond. We feel connected; we understand one another on a much deeper level than most. I meet some incredible and beautiful people during my time at cardiac rehabilitation, both staff members and patients.

Lisa, the registered nurse who provides orientation, guides me for the first couple of sessions. I feel very comfortable with Lisa. One day I ask to speak with her in private. I explain to that outside of class, when I am home, I get feelings of depression and I do not know how to deal with them or what to do. She leaves me momentarily, returning with a book that talks about the depression post-op cardiac patients can experience. She hugs me while telling me that the emotions I feel are natural and that I should not be ashamed. She encourages me to read the book and seek her out any time I would like to discuss it further. Her little act of listening, taking an interest in me, and handing me a helpful tool makes a lasting impression on me, and it demonstrates once again that people do care and want to help.

In some ways, I feel undeserving of the continual gifts I receive from others. The kindness Lisa extends by listening, patting me on the back, and offering a resource is cause for me to think about the impact of the selfless little things that occur all around me.

I will never forget the day I tried to pull a practical joke on Lisa. I am on the treadmill, walking at my usual pace. I spot Lisa sitting at the master console, reviewing everyone's EKG signals while enjoying her morning cup of coffee. I want to know what will happen if I pick up my pace. Just as I notice Lisa looking down at her monitor, I crank up the machine to the point that I have to run to stay on it. Instantly, Lisa spots something on the screen that catches her attention. She is locked in on what is happening. In what seems to be only a couple seconds later, Lisa abruptly looks up, staring intently at me. I look back as if to ask if I am okay to do this. She looks at the monitor then back up at me and, with a smile, gives me a thumbs-up of approval. I soon have to slow the machine down because I am out of breath. But I will never forget witnessing Lisa's deep concern, followed by that smile and her encouraging thumbs-up gesture. Lisa made a lasting impression on me.

Pat is another cardiac care registered nurse, just like Lisa. The word among my fellow patients is that she has a keen eye and can spot trouble in the making with a patient. On one occasion, I saw

Pat approach a patient on the elliptical machine and ask him to stop the exercise. The next thing I know, she is escorting him out of the room. Although I am not sure, I heard a rumor that he has atrial fibrillation and did not know it. Atrial fibrillation is an irregular and often rapid heart rate that can increase the risk of stroke, heart failure, and other heart-related complications. I recall Pat sensing something was wrong even though she was not in front of the master console looking at EKGs. With only her senses, she was able to attend to him. From that point on, I would observe Pat in action. Like a hawk, she continually scans the rooms and checks in on the patients. She makes us all feel safe.

Kellea and Kearci are both exercise physiologists. Humility, leadership, knowledge, experience, and focus are what come to mind when I think of these ladies. It is an honor and privilege to have them work with me during cardiac rehabilitation. I am impressed by their attention to detail and relentless pursuit to have their patients' well-being as their number one priority. And they never complete a sentence without kind and gentle smiles.

Kellea is the one I prefer check my blood pressure before each workout. She always makes a point of smiling at me and saying, "You are good to go!" with an upbeat tone. Often Kellea comes over to where I am working out to ask if I am okay or if I need anything. She never leaves my station without providing words of encouragement or complimenting my progress. The phrase "keep up the good work" is a powerful one I hear her say often. She makes a lasting impression on me with her encouragement and a very positive approach to her work.

Kearci is assigned to me the day I graduate from rehab. Not only is she able to explain my progress, but she also does so in a way that I can fully understand. She motivates me to work hard and carry forward with my cardio regimen well beyond the rehabilitation program. Kearci is a world-ranked professional triathlete. I believe her advanced level of athleticism proves to be a unique advantage in dealing with patients.

I first meet Dan one morning while several of us are in the lobby waiting for our class to begin. Dan and I were blessed with extended life at the same time, as a result of the same surgery. Dan has an attractive personality, engages well in conversation, and is incredibly polite to everyone he meets. I think I might enjoy being his friend. One day, Dan is right in front of me as we check in for class. I overhear Dan giving March 28 as his birthday. I thought he was playing a practical joke on me—that is my birthday! It turns out we have the same birthday. From that moment forward, we begin to form a close bond. We visit before and after class, we catch each other's eye while we are working out and exchange smiles, and we both try to lighten up the mood in class, saying or doing silly things.

I look forward to attending class to spend time with Dan.

When Dan and I are together, we talk about life, family, health, aspirations, and how we want to leave a mark on this world. We talk about the playful times in class, how the staff lifts our spirits, and we even tease each other about who starts and completes the exercises stations the fastest. We also play a game that involves guessing which staff member will check our blood pressure throughout the class.

I am grateful for the opportunity to meet Dan and become friends. Our friendship is best described as two grown men smiling and laughing who share life's experiences with each another, and, in doing so, strengthen their bond of friendship each time they meet.

Throughout my program, it never appears that rehab is just a job for the staff as they freely—and with a smile—use their skills, talent, confidence, and approach to provide a new life for each of their patients.

I put a name to this new life: Life 2.0.

During each session, I begin with my third station: the recumbent bicycle. At the same time, a classmate starts the arm pedal exerciser. I gather she is in bad shape and has several things wrong with her heart. I never see her smile and think she is deeply depressed and saddened by life. By far, she is the most introverted and quiet patient in the class. She pretty much stays to herself. One day, while feeling guilty about the amount of love, attention, and guidance I have been receiving, I decide that maybe I should pass some on to this other patient. I make it a goal to get her to smile, something I have not seen her do since we met. At first, we chitchat about the class and exercise in general. Eventually, the topics spread to other things, like the local news. One day I tell her how much I admire her efforts to attend class and put forth the effort to improve her health. She cracks a little smile and whispers, "Thank you."

I have worked hard to get her to smile; it is so crucial for me to give her a moment of peace and happiness, which she deserves to experience. From that day forward, she is more and more friendly to me and produces a smile as we work out and converse. I believe she feels safe with me, and because I acknowledge her existence, she is driven to improve. I wonder if I have made a lasting impression on her. I want her to experience that just as I have experienced lasting impressions from others.

Just after my heart catheterization procedure, I wrote a letter to the hospital praising them for the people they employ and telling them how I enjoyed an exceptional experience during a time I needed help. In closing, I offered to help them with anything they would like me to do. That offer led to an opportunity to meet Brien, a marketing manager for the hospital. One day during class, I am on the treadmill, almost out of breath and looking forward to being done. I look up and see a man standing in front of my machine, looking at me and smiling.

"You must be Kevin. I am Brien. Nice to meet you," he says. When my workout is complete, he tells me there are opportunities for me to participate in their marketing program and they like to use real-life patients for testimonials and other related activities. I am thrilled to have the opportunity to help. I do not know at the time that my decision to help would profoundly benefit others and, in some cases, would save and restore lives.

I am now only a few sessions away from graduation day for a class that has been life-changing for me. The course has taught me the importance of activity, exercise, nutrition, and personal inspiration. Just 150 minutes per week makes a difference. After class graduation, I am planning to walk more, take stairs instead of elevators, and park farther away from the store. Every step counts.

I also plan to eat better, focusing on lean meats, fish, and lots of veggies. I want to get serious about my heart and overall physical condition. I learn it is important to limit sugar and salt while opting for heart-healthy fats like avocado and olive oil. The staff, especially Lisa, helps me understand that heart health isn't just about veins and arteries; it is also about my emotional well-being and stress management. Taking a few minutes to meditate or doing some deep breathing exercises every day to manage stress is very beneficial.

The big day—graduation—arrives. This makes me both excited and sad. I am thrilled to have learned a lot from the rehabilitation program, the other people, and myself. I experience a feeling of sadness, and I am sorry to leave. I feel attached, somewhat dependent, on being monitored and cared for each day.

I am looking forward to getting my last smile and wave from the lady at the emergency room desk and participating in my graduation ceremony in which they will play "Pomp and Circumstance," a famous piece of music played at formal services.

Heading from my car to the emergency room door, I think, "This may be the last smile and wave I get from the lady behind the desk; I sure hope she is there today. Oh good, I can see her as I walk in the door." I begin to smile and prepare to wave as she turns her head toward me. For a moment, I feel stunned. That same spiritual presence as the woman I saw the last day of my hospital stay permeates from the eyes of this lady. I feel so loved and safe as her smile radiates throughout the hallway and she provides that ever so familiar wave.

What did I see?

I must go meet her, talk to her, and thank her for the comfort she brings me every time I walk past her. Suddenly I hear the door to the class open and the staff is calling us to come in and get started. I turn and walk toward class, knowing I will see this lady after class.

Today, Kearci is assigned to record my final results, help me interpret them, and answer any questions I have about my routines and exercise beyond the class. She takes blood pressure readings at various stages of my workout. As she does, she continually offers words of encouragement and expresses that she is proud of me and the things I have accomplished.

When the workouts are complete and the scores are recorded, they start the "Pomp and Circumstance" music. So many of my classmates congratulate me and wish me the very best as we say goodbye. It feels bittersweet.

Although the staff reports I have made good progress and finished the program well, they have no idea just how well I finish until I gather them at the conclusion of my last exercise station. Once my graduation picture is taken with the staff by my side, I ask for a minute of their time so that I can share something with them. I've included what I share below.

"I did not choose to be here, but I am. You do not know this, but at one point in my life, I am a finely tuned collegiate athlete and throughout the years, made some poor choices in my lifestyle. Although recovery has been a challenge, you were not aware of how well I disguised the mentally and emotionally dark and depressing places I found myself in. It began with thoughts of 'why me, how much longer do I have, is my life coming to an end.' Your knowledge and training have given me confidence and the tools to carry on my life. Your encouragement gives me hope. Most remarkable, your attitude and approach to your care provide me with life, so bless you, and thank you. You, fine people, are not working a job and collecting a paycheck, you are changing lives, just like so many associated with this hospital. I do

not believe I could have escaped the dark places on my own, because of you I did. Every day you give me a helping hand, a smile, some encouragement, and a feeling that I am important, you are here for me. Not once do I observe any of you are tired, disinterested, distracted, or otherwise "not into it," but yet it was 6:30 in the morning. Your passion, work ethic, and teamwork aimed at helping others indeed led me to a monumental discovery, the discovery of a miracle, the miracle of experiencing life unlike I have ever felt it before. My outlook on life is exponentially more powerful and positive than ever before, and I find it challenging to find the words to describe it. Those in my circle know me as a very positive influence. Until now, I have had no idea the degree to which I could be happy, positive, confident, desirous to help others, and, most of all, humble and appreciative. You are the icing on the cake of my life."

There are far more strangers in this world than people we know. I too am a stranger to millions of people, but oh how good and connected I feel when one of them expresses an interest in me, my well-being, my successes, my failures, and my priorities. I recall a conversation with Susan, the chief nursing officer, some time ago. I was quizzing her about her approach to making sure patients feel important, well-regarded, and cared for by the nursing team. Her reply is, "I ask that my nurses learn something about each of their patients that us not in their chart and build on that."

Every patient in my class was once a stranger.

Time changed that.

I remember meeting Dan, who, to this day, is a terrific friend of mine. We see each other regularly.

I recall the lady exercising next to me, cracking a smile after I say something to her. Sadly, I only saw her smile a few times.

I remember the guy who appears to be the popular one, the one who seems to have it all together. On the surface, he looks confident, yet, in the parking lot, we would talk about our fears, our outlooks on life, and our sadness over the condition we found ourselves in. We would end each conversation with a smile and a handshake. It felt right; it felt warm; it's still with me.

I remember the large, muscular man, who, as a stranger, looked confident and in control of his surroundings, like he didn't need any help. However, as I got to know him, I learn he is scared and in need of companionship.

I remember the guy who continued to have problems with his heart. We would talk about it before class. I could tell he found comfort in his classmates' interest in him. I always found a way to catch his eye in class and give a quick wave and a smile, getting one back in return.

I remember the quiet man. He did not talk to anyone except the staff, choosing to keep to himself. I approached him the day he graduated, hugged him, congratulated him, and let him know I admired him, so much so that I try to model my work ethic after his. He said, "That means a lot to me. Thank you for telling me that." We gripped each other's hands and, in that moment, knew we were no longer strangers. We made a difference to one another. Those are the only words I ever heard him speak; yet, it is as beautiful and vivid to me today as it was then.

We were all connected, no longer strangers. Our rehabilitation went well beyond the physical.

I am motivated to add positivity to the lives of others because that is what the rehabilitation team and my classmates did for me. They made a difference, and I am honored to know them and humbled by their giving and caring ways.

Chapter 11:

Daily choice – Live or die?

*n*ow what? Having survived surgery and completed cardiac rehabilitation, I contemplate what to do.

Where do I go from here?

I'm still alive…what now?

There are no more nurses looking after me, there is no more EKG monitoring during rehabilitation workouts, no more intensive medical care and attention.

What I do know is that healthcare professionals inspire me. They are just like me. They have bills to pay, spouses, children, ups, downs, and all the same issues in life. Yet they give and give and give and give and ask for nothing in return. They are selflessly dedicating their time, energy, and talent to better the likes of people like me.

One day, as I quietly think about my life, my future, and my mortality, I realize it is time to start taking my health more seriously. It is time to take control. With so many experts available to help me, why would I not want to become an expert in my own health?

I must learn how to eat, how to exercise, and how to take my medications. Working to reduce the risk of a heart attack or stroke must become a way of life for me. I have enjoyed thirty-four years of marriage with June. What is required to get another thirty-four years with her?

I come to grips with the fact that lifestyle changes, in paramount proportions, are in store for me. However, how do I go about those changes?

Thinking back to the time I learned the frightening news that my next step might be my last, I remember going immediately into survival mode.

That's it!

I must wake up every day and answer this question before I get started: live or die? Do I choose to prolong or shorten my life? If I choose to die, there is no work for me to do. If I choose to live, I must, every day, be disciplined enough to exercise, eat correctly, take my medications, and connect with my spirituality. I must answer this same question each day for the remainder of my life.

Live or die?

I decide that I need to have a baseline and targets for things like cholesterol, blood sugar, and my weight, so that I can monitor my progress and results. I write down cholesterol targets, which I will track every time I have bloodwork done. I design a daily and twice-daily cardiac exercise program, based in large part on what

I learned in rehabilitation. I study books on diabetic dieting. I prepare meal plan options that I can choose from to supplement my daily exercise regimen.

What begins to unfold is a more profound sense of—and commitment to—my new and beautiful life: Life 2.0. This is an experience I want to cling to as I age. I attribute this new life to the ways and the teachings of the healthcare providers, both clinical and not clinical, that touched my family and me. I went through this transformation primarily after being inspired by the unconditional giving from all levels and functions within the medical community. Their giving motivates me to give back, to show them what is truly possible, to remind them of their relevance, their importance, and their value—and to make sure they know they are never forgotten.

What happens when we receive bad news? How do we cope with and internalize it? What goes on between doctor and patient, patient and family? What do the nurses and supporting staff face? Learning the answers to these questions requires a personal understanding of the patient. Would it be helpful for our future nurses to know that even just providing simple, straightforward, caring practices can shape lives in ways far beyond the imagination?

Opportunities to remind caregivers and the surrounding support staff that they will never be forgotten are the most rewarding opportunities for me. These wonderful healthcare professionals should never be left behind. Caregivers and support staff need to know how significant they are to patients, their families, and their loved ones. They need help recognizing newer and higher possibilities for their lives. What was done for my family and me gives me a deep desire to show healthcare professionals their value.

If they can give, so can I.

Making a daily choice to live or die becomes my foundation for living with cardiovascular disease and my motivation to pay it forward by positively impacting the lives of others. I commit to making daily choices in these three categories to prolong my life:

- Diet discipline
- Exercise habit
- Medication regimen

Given that this will be a lot of work, I wonder how I can discipline myself to stay with it. The answer for me is to make it fun. I create a game for my activities. For example, I learn that exercising would lower my blood sugar, hence the cardiac rehabilitation staff's insistence that my blood sugar is at a certain threshold before exercise. A few times, I test my blood sugar immediately following a workout. My results are consistently lower than before exercising. The game I create is to see how many blood sugar points I can drop in twenty minutes of exercise, forty minutes of exercise, and sixty minutes of exercise. I usually try to beat my previous time. To do that, I have to work out harder than the previous time. I also vary the types and quantities of food intake before a workout so I can learn what impact food has on my blood sugar reduction—if any.

Step by step, I work to reduce my risk of a heart attack or stroke. And my results begin to improve. In just six months I:

- Form a cardio daily exercise habit
- Lose fifty pounds
- Achieve excellent vital statistics
- Beat diabetes (my doctor took me off medication)
- Learn more about Life 2.0

Even though the physical element of my life improves immensely, I am more drawn to my spirituality, my belief, and my faith in God. After all, I was on the road to death. Why was my life spared? Why were so many people instrumental, putting their lives on hold for me? Why did I feel such a profound impact on my experience from observing others doing simple and little things? Why did the Angels appear to me? There must be something more; I must have a purpose.

Although I do not know what my purpose is, or what I am to focus on in this new life, I commit to opening my eyes and ears so that when it is revealed to me, I won't miss it.

I evolve from experiencing an intense scare to a daily practice of survival. I ask myself why I chose to live in response to the daily question "live or die." Throughout most of my life, I have chosen "live," primarily because I was afraid to die. I never wanted to die; I never looked forward to it; I was scared of it.

While I was attending cardiac rehabilitation, I felt as though my life were going through a transformation. I did not question it; I did not fight it. I began accepting, endorsing, and welcoming those feelings. I wanted to learn more, to feel more, to understand where those feelings were taking me. I wanted to know if this was the beginning of understanding my purpose.

What unfolded is an unparalleled transformation to living life differently, living with new focus and priorities. How I see others, and the importance of putting myself in a position to impact others, becomes the cornerstone of my daily interests.

I believe this transformation was sparked while I was being cared for in the hospital. It was cemented by God—beginning with His revelation of Angels.

Chapter 12:

The Angels that walk among us

As a child, I learned about Angels in church. From my best recollection (and from pictures on the internet), they are presented with wings, sometime wearing halos, and often flying around playing a harp.

I believe Angels have many distinct qualities:

- Indirect: We see the work they do without seeing them directly
- Quiet: They are unassuming and do not seek attention
- Nurturing: They comfort us in times of need
- Protecting: They protect us from evil forces
- Guiding: They help guide our lives and our paths

- Unselfish: They are present to serve, guide, and shelter, asking nothing in return

In my experiences, I have had a few questions I am unable to answer.

What made me ask my doctor the question that saved my life?

Why am I so attune with the little things people do? Why can I observe how significantly they impact lives?

Why do I feel as though I must have a purpose? And why do I feel a sense of urgency to find that purpose?

I now know that divine intervention takes place in my life. I no longer fear death. I am at peace. I have learned how to improve myself so that I can see the good in all situations, as well as the good in all people through the little things they do. In turn, I can pay it forward with the little things I do.

I do not ask for divine intervention, and I do not think about it. It just happens. Angels appear to me on three separate occasions. I am not sure if there is significance in the number three. I do not see wings, I do not see harps, and I do not see any of them floating in space. What I do see and experience, within my soul, can only be described as beautiful, peaceful, and filled with love, compassion, and protection. In each of the three instances, the experience lasts for only a few fleeting moments.

I believe Angels have been carrying me, caring for me, and guiding me…but why? Why are my eyes, ears, and heart suddenly open, taking in new observations about the world around me in ways I have never before?

The Angels are speaking to me; they do indeed walk among us. I saw them through the eyes of ordinary, everyday people.

As I described earlier, the Angel experience occurs during my release from the hospital. My discharge paperwork is complete, my belongings are packed, and I am placed in a wheelchair, which will be used to transport me to our car. As I wheel toward the elevators, we pass by the nursing station. I notice several nurses smiling at me; they know I am happy to be going home. I remember raising my arm and somewhat loudly proclaiming my thanks to the nurses for saving my life. As I say the word "life," something far to my left on the other side of the nursing station catches my attention. As I sharply turn to look, I see a nurse walking in the opposite direction down the hall. She is smiling, looking right at me as she continues to walk. During the split second I see her, I notice something incredibly special in her eyes, something warm, reassuring, protective, compassionate, and deeply loving. Never before have I experienced anything like this. I can only describe what I see as amazingly Angelic. As she rounds the corner and disappears from my sight, I immediately think, "I just saw an Angel."

Could this be true?

Probably not. After all, she did not have wings, was not wearing a heavenly robe, and was not toting a harp. But I do have a sense of being genuinely cared for and watched over. I do feel love and acknowledgment, which soothes me and lifts me spiritually. I don't say another word as I leave the hospital and approach our car, where June is waiting for me. I am just not sure what to say.

Riding in a car for the first time after surgery is challenging. Even though I feel some pain in my chest area, it is nothing compared to the anxiety of what will happen if we hit a bump, or if my wife must hit the brakes hard. During the ride, all I can do is think about seeing the Angel. The challenges of riding in the car faded in comparison to the thoughts about what I saw. I do not want to come across as crazy, so I refrain from talking about it with anyone other than with June. To this day, I recall that moment as if it just happened seconds ago.

The next time an Angel is revealed is on my graduation day from rehabilitation. Again, this is also described in an earlier chapter. Routinely, on days I attend rehab, I park in the emergency room parking lot, walk through the emergency room doors, and walk down a hallway to the entryway to rehab. During that short walk, I would pass by a glass-enclosed office. I believe that is where patients check in when visiting the emergency room. Before every rehab session, at approximately 6:15 a.m., I walk by that office and catch a glimpse of the lady sitting at the desk. She gives me a friendly smile; I enjoy that. Her smile eventually turns into a smile plus a wave. I do not know her; however, I find myself looking forward to seeing her and getting the smile and wave she generously gives to me each time. Finally, graduation day arrives. As I drive to class, I can't help but feel sad about this being the last day I will see the caring specialists, my classmates, and the smile and wave from the emergency room attendant.

As usual, I enter the doors to the emergency room, and as I approach the office where the attendant sits, she looks at me and extends her familiar smile and wave. I experience the same sensation looking into her eyes as I did the day I was released from the hospital. In those few moments, I see and experience a love that deeply consumes me, a feeling of overabundant caring and watchfulness over me. Even though I am walking, it feels as though I am perfectly still, absorbing the moment in its entirety. Indeed, I see an Angel.

Do I mention it to anyone, or will they think something is wrong with me?

I decide I am going to introduce myself to this lady. I want to meet her; I have to meet her. Suddenly, I hear the rehab door open and the familiar voice instructing all of us to enter and get prepared for class. I decide I will see the lady and introduce myself immediately after class.

After class, I promptly return to the ER to meet her…but she is not there. I learn she works the night shift and leaves by 7 a.m.

A month later, I rise early and head to the hospital to meet her. I explain to her the significance and importance of her role, as simple as it seems, in my recovery and how having something to look forward to makes a huge difference, even if it involves people we have not met. I can tell she is genuinely appreciative and happy that she made an impact on my life. She looks like an ordinary person that day, just like she did every time I saw her. No signs of an Angel this time.

A few months after my graduation from rehabilitation, I attend a men's health event, hosted by the heart hospital. As I am leaving, I make my way toward the main hospital revolving glass door. As I approach the door, I notice a rather large man at the door, on his hands and knees, washing the glass with his back to me. When I get closer, I say, "You are doing a great job. I promise not to mess it up as I leave."

As I say this, he is getting up. He turns toward me and, with smile that would warm anyone's heart, replies, "It's alright if you do so sir."

What man, after working hard to clean windows on his hands and knees, would be so gracious as to tell a stranger it was okay to ruin the work he was doing, and give off the impression he would be happy to clean it up again and again? As I glance at his face, I see an Angel through his eyes, which envelopes me with an extraordinary feeling of love, protection, and peace. That moment then transitions to me shaking the hand of this special man who presents an Angel to me. I did not tell him what I experienced—it feels so private, so reassuring, so spiritual.

At this point, without a doubt, I know there is something I must do in this world…but what? How to do I find out what my purpose is? My eyes, ears, and heart must be fully open to accept my purpose, my role in this world.

The man's who is washing the glass that day is Alvin, and he is the same man who came into room 610 to clean on my first day in the hospital after my surgery. Eventually, I decide to write him a letter, compelled to share my experience.

Hello Alvin,

For many months, I have meant to reach out to you. Why? Believe it or not, you have played a pivotal and profound role in my life. You and I first encountered one another in 2014, in the lobby of the hospital during a community event. It was during that brief encounter with you that my perspective on life completely changed. I have shared the experience with many people all around the world. It is with great humility and gratitude that I share it with the most important character in this story, you.

In February of last year, Dr. Moore performed open-heart surgery on me at your hospital. I made an excellent recovery from the surgery and improved my health substantially as a result of your fabulous rehabilitation team, but more importantly, because of the very genuine, kind, compassionate, and caring people from every aspect of the hospital, with you being on the center stage of that.

You see, Alvin, during my recovery, I must admit I became depressed. I felt defeated and continually fought to produce a positive attitude. I needed to accept my condition as a blessing, a blessing that I could spend more time with my wife, and my family, something I believe to be the most essential part of my life.

One day, while walking out of the hospital, there was a man on his hands and knees, at the main door, wiping something off the floor and cleaning the base of the revolving glass door. Perhaps somebody had spilled something, but it was evident as I approached this man, he was working hard to clean it up. As I approached, and as I neared, I said: "You are doing a great job, I promise not to mess it up as I leave." This man stood up, and as he turned towards me, he said with a big smile, "It's quite all right if you do, sir." First of all, I was stunned by what he said. What man, I thought, after working very hard on something, would be so gracious as to tell a stranger that it was okay to ruin the work he was doing and give the impression he would be happy to clean it up again, and again. I have not shared this next part with many people. I have also been blessed by Angels, and have seen Angels through the eyes of people on three occasions since my surgery. That day was the third time, and it was through the eyes of this man I saw an Angel. Alvin, that man was you.

As I left the building, I realized I was doing everything medical science tells me to do, to live as long and healthy as I can. I recognized that my real job is to rid myself of any apprehension about dying and to live my days out by honoring others, being kind to others, including strangers, and giving back as much as I can to those who paved the way for me. I have given this life a name: I call it Life 2.0.

Since that pivotal day in the hospital, you and I met again. It was during the annual Employee Awards Banquet, where I was given the most incredible honor by Mark Valentine to be your guest speaker. During that evening, I made a point to find a way to shake your hand, and I did. Although I was not able to share this intimate story with you during that festive evening, I want you to know that meeting you again was a significant highlight. The topic I spoke about was, "As patients, we move on, we move forward, but we never forget...We never forget the little things." Alvin, while on that stage, giving that speech, I was hoping you were out there, wishing you could hear me speak, hoping you could listen to how the little things matter. I was so happy to find out later that indeed you were there.

During the speech that night I said: "Our surgeons hold our hearts in their hands, and then restart them, you hold our lives in your hearts, and then you restart them, mold them, contour and shape them in such a manner I never thought possible or imagined." You are a perfect example of that; you had no idea how profoundly our encounter has impacted my life and will continue to forever.

There are no words that can adequately thank you for the gift of Life 2.0, which you contributed to creating for me. I am profoundly grateful and honored to have experienced a part of you, Alvin. Thank you for showing me your kindness, and showing how the "little things" really make a difference. I pray the Angels will appear in your life as they have in mine.

If you ever hear a story about the guy who calls your hospital "The Hospital of Angels," you will know who he is and why he says that and that you are a part of it.

May God eternally bless you, Alvin.

Sincerely,
Kevin Kirksey
a.k.a. K2.0

I learned, much later, that Alvin was a deacon at his church. I learned this at his funeral; he passed away less than a year after I connected with him. He will always be in my heart—and so will the Angel revealed in Alvin's eyes.

I feel some reassurance that now is not my time to leave this earth. I now believe there is meaning and purpose to my life—a plan. I hope to learn what that is very soon, or perhaps I am meant to understand my purpose later in life or even beyond this life.

I have come to believe the Angels represent a safe place, an understanding, a support system, a place of encouragement, of solidarity, of love, of peace. Their purpose is to shine a guiding light on the miracle of life.

The Angels, indeed, walk among us.

Chapter 13:
Life 2.0

This chapter is dedicated to sharing my perspective of Life 2.0 and the things I have learned in hopes that others are inspired to create their own Life 2.0. Life 2.0 is very personal, and it's intended for anyone who wants to live it. Although it is a gift made available by God, each person must make a daily choice to receive that gift.

If I were given a choice between the few short years since my life-saving surgery—during the time God opens my eyes, ears, and heart to Life 2.0—and the fifty-seven years before my surgery, I would choose the few short years every time. My life has been restored, extended, and enhanced in ways I never thought possible—physically, mentally, emotionally, and spiritually.

The premise of Life 2.0 is our ability to separate the actions and unfamiliarity of others from their innate value as human beings. To affirm someone's relevance and importance by demonstrating their value is a form of love that each of us has available to give. Life 2.0 has taught me that this form of love breathes life into people.

Think about it. Telling someone how important they are and emphasizing what a difference they make ignites their feelings of worth as a human being. Since life was given to me, I feel compelled to contribute to bringing life to others by affirming their value, worth, importance, and relevance—things God has shown me that every human, regardless of their actions, deserves.

Earlier, I talked about my classmates in rehab no longer being strangers. In this chapter, as one of Life 2.0's core principles, I claim there is no such thing as a stranger in this world. The concept of "nobody is a stranger" is core in living Life 2.0.

How does one accurately describe moving from a point in a life that contains doubt, anxiety, and depression to a new and beautiful life void of these things? Phrases like "transformation" and "new awakening" come to mind. But Life 2.0 is the term I use to frame this transformation, a term that shines a bright light on what I should focus on instead of the darkness preventing me from seeing God's wishes.

Having a new perspective on life, influenced by whispers from God, opens my eyes, ears, and heart to see and love the world from the standpoints of others versus my own standpoint. A countless number of tireless healthcare workers exposed God's gift of Life 2.0 to me, and for that, I am eternally grateful. I have something below I would like to tell every person in healthcare. If I could pray these words on a piece of paper and place that piece of paper in their pockets or under their pillows at night, I would.

> *"As patients, we move on, we move forward, but we never forget. You are never left behind, especially in our prayers. Your inspiration, love, compassion, humility, and kindness illuminate the little things you do, making lasting impressions and planting the seed of Life 2.0.*
>
> *In the operating room, our surgeons hold our hearts in their hands and restart them. In the operating room of life, healthcare workers hold our lives in their hearts and restart them, shape them, and mold them in ways patients might never think possible — physically, emotionally, and spiritually."*

In my case, a simple question and an inexpensive test not only save my life but also are the catalysts for me to awaken into this new life and proceed on a journey filled with opportunity to impact the experiences of others. I am eternally grateful for this gift from God.

So, how did Life 2.0 begin?

Life 2.0 is born during my stay in room 610 at the hospital and continues to grow and blossom. Before this period of my life, I was living a life—let's call it Life 1.0—all about me: my life, what I need, what I want. In some ways, that life was selfish. Life 2.0, on the other hand, is about the lives of others and how I can contribute something positive to their lives, no matter how small or insignificant, and perhaps inspire them in some small—or profound—way.

As I look back, beginning when I learned my life was in danger through the point I am fully restored, I am reminded of the parable about the mustard seed. In the Gospel of Matthew, (Matthew 12:31-32, World English Bible) the parable is as follows:

> *He set another man before them, saying, "The Kingdom of Heaven is like a grain of mustard seed, which a man took, and sowed in his field; which indeed is smaller than all seeds. But when it is grown, it is greater than the herbs and becomes a tree so that the birds of the air come and lodge in its branches."*

I now realize my inspiration for living Life 2.0 comes from observing others and listening for God's whispers. My eyes, ears, and heart are open to the world around me, whereas before they were not.

Think about it. So many of the people we encounter each day are strangers. They surround us; they show up in every facet of our daily living. We see hundreds of them every day. We can't escape strangers. We see them at work, in the grocery store, at a restaurant, on the highways, on airplanes, just about everywhere we find ourselves throughout our days. We look at their faces, which are often mirrors revealing something about them. As I pondered the enormous number of strangers in this world, I realized that I too was a stranger to millions of people. And I felt so alive and connected when one of those strangers expressed an interest in my well-being, my successes, my failures, and my priorities—when they expressed an interest in me as a human.

Are they indeed strangers?

I used to think so.

But I have realized that those we believe are strangers…are not.

Instead, they are friends. Everyone lives with pain, personal demons, and challenges in their life. These come in varying forms and degrees of magnitude, e.g., illness, betrayal, financial ruin, career disappointment, loneliness, depression, spiritually broken heart. These are just to name a few. When we see a person, a stranger, most often, we do not know what burdens they carry in life. The Angels showed me, through the eyes of others and the little things others do, an unconditional love, a love that I feel called to pass on to everyone I encounter. To do that, I must approach my life and everyone around me differently, hence the label Life 2.0. The true essence of Life 2.0 is not about me; it's about what I can do for others by trying to see the world from their perspective and be a friend to everyone. By doing so, I remove all strangers in my life.

If we label someone a stranger, it is because we are not able to assign value to their existence or we are not ready and willing to open our hearts to them. Those who cared for me, both directly and indirectly, including the Angels, expose Life 2.0 to me in a way that feels spiritually grounded, thereby offering me an invitation to live it. The world is so much better as we tap into the lives of others through little things we do and offer expressions of compassion, empathy, and humility. Everyone deserves to feel relevant and valuable. We are all God's children, and no one has to be labeled a stranger.

We all understand that life can be a burden at times. It often includes frustration, doubt, uncertainty, sadness, and other things that consume us and get in our way. Everyone who was involved in some fashion of my care put their life on hold so that I could further enjoy my loved ones, spend more time with my friends, and continue to pursue my dreams.

Perhaps there are now things I can give back. Is it possible that I can give back in the same way they gave to me? After all, life presents its burdens to everyone, including those directly or indirectly involved in my care. Those individuals deserve to be reminded of the great work they do for others by saving, restoring, extending, and enhancing life. Doesn't everyone in the world deserve to be acknowledged for the great work they do, no matter what it is?

It soon became apparent to me that acknowledgment, kindness, thankfulness, and recognition, even in the smallest doses, can have a far-reaching impact on the lives of others.

So, how did it all begin to unfold?

Little by little, I began to notice little things occurring around me, starting with the people working tirelessly and selflessly to help and support me and the other patients. They live with their own set of life's challenges, but they prioritized taking care of others, including me, ahead of themselves.

Perhaps there is a better way to live.

I have counted over 120 little things I observed in others that inspired me to lead a new life. The foundation of Life 2.0 is built of many little things that make lasting impressions, just simple encounters with others.

I experience a nurse, Editha, who makes a game out of who could most accurately guess my blood sugar readings every hour. At the time, I did not realize what she was doing by playing this game with me. She is purposeful, thoughtful, and kind by giving me a mental break from the pain. She doesn't have to do this. She offers this little thing, our game, for my benefit.

I notice a lady sitting at a desk behind a glass window in the emergency room. She offers a smile to me every day as I walk past her office on my way to rehabilitation class. Those smiles turn into both a smile and a wave. I believe she knows a smile is a gift to a patient like me, as she gives it so freely, so effortlessly, despite her burdens. Even today, I am inspired by her selfless act of kindness and motivated to pass it on some way, somehow.

I learn of a security guard being compassionate and kind to my wife, ministering to her when I could not. He did not need to do that. He did so because he possesses compassion and chose to use it in a simple, yet profound, way.

On the day of my surgery, a warm blanket was placed over me before I was taken to the operating room. I remember thinking that there is a person in the hospital who gathers, washes, and organizes those blankets so that people like me can be comfortable. Even though I was heading to surgery, not knowing if I would see my wife again, I held on to a desire to one day find this person and thank them for making an impact, for making a stressful situation a little bit better, for me, a stranger. I want this person to know that their work behind the scenes is recognized and appreciated. Months later, I made an effort to locate and meet this person. Her name is Kristie. I let her know that even though we never had any direct contact, she touched my life in a positive, warm, and caring way.

I remember walking around the nurse's station, for the very first time after surgery, and receiving a high five from a nurse, Beth, for this accomplishment. I didn't get a job promotion; I didn't win the lottery; I didn't win an award. All I did was walk around a nurse's station. That little thing, the high five, becomes the catalyst for my rapid recovery, earning me the nickname "Rock Star."

I observe a large number of supplies, linens, and other items used to care for me. Somewhere in the system is a person responsible for ordering those supplies and staying on top of inventory so that there is enough for everyone. What an important role they play. I can only imagine the person performing these duties behind the scenes does not know how appreciated they are and what a significant role they play in the well-being of the patient.

A year after surgery, while standing in the lobby of the hospital, I watch a team of surgical nurses walk by. One of them stopped, approached me, smiled, and said, "I remember you. How are you?" I immediately feel relevant and valued, just hearing, "I remember you."

Roy, one of the nurses not assigned to me, visited my room to help out during a busy day on the floor. He stayed a few extra minutes to help me with my breathing, show me how to get up and down, and visit with me for a moment. Roy is very busy but takes time to demonstrate how important I am just by sitting with me, talking, and helping me improve my breathing, even though he is not required to do so.

One day, the chief nursing officer, Susan, shares her belief in the importance of her staff learning something about each patient that is not in their chart. That is such a little thing to do; however, acknowledging a patient in this way validates their value and importance and pays tribute to them as a human being. I can only imagine how significant that can be for a patient coming into the system who is not feeling valuable or worthy.

As I write this book, I yearn to connect with people and remind them of the excellent work they do by demonstrating to them how far-reaching a little thing can be. I want everyone to be blessed with feelings of pride, relevance, and importance. I want everyone to be allowed to see how good an outcome can be and how they contribute to those outcomes through the little things they do.

Life 2.0 is a miraculous journey—one I credit the nurses and their noble profession for as they put me on the path to experience it. Although it is seen as just a "little thing," I am infinitely thankful to them for their dedication and endless pursuit to provide gold-standard care to their patients and the patients' families. I pray that one day, when they need it most, they can feel my encouragement, my acknowledgment, and my appreciation. I hope the Angels carry and care for them as they did me, and, in doing so, touch them with the power of little things.

Healthcare workers inspire me. I realize they are humans just like me; they have bills to pay, spouses, children, and issues in life. At a point in time when this is all beginning to make sense to me, I make a decision to validate as many healthcare workers as I can, enhancing their connection with their higher purpose by expressing my thanks and appreciation in the very best manner I can. Let's face it, we all know about the hard facets of the healthcare profession. It does not always go well. They deal with extraordinarily sick and broken people, surrounded in an emotional pressure cooker every day. The patients who do well, like me, leave the hospital and go on their way. For patients, healthcare workers are never forgotten or left behind, especially in our prayers. Their knowledge, skill, and teamwork give me confidence, their encouragement gives me hope, and their attitude and approach gives me a life to live.

They placed their lives on hold for me. They taught me about my medications and what they do. They taught me how to eat, how to exercise, and how to smile for no reason. They taught me how to be kind to a stranger and how wonderful that can be. They encouraged me, challenged me, and even high fived me. They asked for nothing in return.

That is how I want to be. That is what Life 2.0 tells me to work toward. It's no longer about me; it's about living a life that positively impacts the lives of others through doing little things...and asking for nothing in return.

I am working on getting the maximum I can out of life as a testament to the health profession's attitude that everyone matters, everyone is relevant, and the impact everyone makes on the lives of others is far more significant than easily observed.

Life 2.0 permeates the physical, mental, emotional, and spiritual aspects of life, all in unison. The sum of the little things I experienced helped me realize things about myself—and about life—which would change me forever.

How can I possibly touch the lives of others and give back even a small fraction of what they gave to me? How can I apply my experiences and what I have learned from others and from God to change the course of my life? How can I be the best I can be, not for myself, but for them?

Perhaps God is asking me to step back and hold the door open for my brothers and sisters with the little things others made possible for me to do.

Soon after surgery, I came to realize that if I do everything the medical profession asks me to do, e.g., exercise, eat properly, and take my medications, there is nothing more I can do to control my health, negating the need or temptation to worry. As a result, I am no longer afraid of dying. I am no longer depressed, no longer questioning my longevity. I spend time working on improving myself mentally, physically, emotionally, and spiritually so that I have something to offer others, even if it's just a little thing.

In some ways, Life 2.0 gives me a heightened sense of life—at times, euphoric. I see others like I never did before. And I see Angels through the eyes of others.

After seeing the tireless hours put in by all departments, and the selfless acts of kindness while providing a gold-standard quality of care, I became genuinely motivated to demonstrate that everyone in the healthcare system contributes to saving, restoring, extending, and enhancing life. To do this, I must work at being the best I can be physically, mentally, emotionally, and spiritually. Some of the efforts I have made, and continue to make daily, include:

- **Physically** – I developed a cardio exercise habit seven days per week along with a diet discipline. The results included losing fifty pounds, beating diabetes, and maintaining excellent vitals.

- **Mentally** – I have taught myself to make a game out of my discipline, remembering every day where I came from and what I must do to keep moving forward. In my calendar, at 7 a.m., seven days a week, there is an entry titled "Thanks-4-Giving Day" as a reminder to thank someone for giving to others.

- **Emotionally** – I try to make every situation about others, I try very hard to honor others daily and express humility. Compassion for others is profoundly present in my day-to-day living. Often, I tear up and feel tingling throughout my body when I see a stranger, knowing they are just like me, living the best they can given their surroundings, circumstances, and the cards they are dealt in life. I want them to know they are loved, they are cared for, and Angels are indeed among us.

- **Spiritually** – I have made peace with my Maker because I am doing everything I can for my health. I am not afraid to die. I am loving life. I am at peace. I often pray and listen to God's whispers.

Life 2.0 is available to everyone, not just those who are fortunate enough to be fully recovered from a life-threatening event and living an extended life.

During rehabilitation, I was amongst patients with different conditions, outcomes, and prognoses. Many of these people are working to maximize the physical, mental, and emotional aspects of their situations. At the same time, the rehabilitation staff is investing heavily in each patient to give them the very best chance of success. People are not always who and what they appear to be; they often mask underlying challenges, pain, and dreams in their lives. Life 2.0 compels me to work hard at being kind and understanding to everyone I come in contact with, no matter how big their smile. After all, that smile may very well be a mask.

Most people think of the room where cardiac rehabilitation takes place as a fitness center or exercise facility, spaciously organized and filled with quality equipment. I view it as a place where patients see hope, a new beginning and a place to dream of better days ahead. Perhaps some view it as a ticket to a new and improved life—for themselves, their families, loved ones, and friends.

When I was in rehabilitation, it was never about the exercise routine at all. The value for me was in how the workers supported me and built my confidence in my ability to do everything. They helped convince me that I can succeed, and I can live life. I view them as compassionate, loving, accommodating, and skilled people, who selflessly work extremely hard to improve lives, and they do so with the patience of Angels. They taught me how to improve my heart function, and in doing so, occupy a special place in my heart forever.

I believe all big things in life are created with the summation of little things. If I can offer little things to those around me, perhaps I can contribute to something big in their life, something that God whispers to me to do, something that makes the Angels smile.

I have learned that the blessings in our lives are formed by those around us—including strangers.

I envision living Life 2.0 for the remainder of my years. It is not a one-time thing; it's a journey forward, a lifestyle. There is no reason for me not be the best I can be for the benefit of others, no matter the situation or circumstance.

God put me on a path to a new life I never imagined possible. He has helped me open my eyes, ears, and heart to living a life focused on others versus myself. The new normal of waking each day excited by the opportunity to delight someone else is spiritually pleasurable. I believe I am now aging as a happier, kinder, sweeter person. Based on my experiences, I believe Life 2.0 is a gift available to everyone, regardless of situation, affliction, or circumstance. All we have to do is choose to live it each day.

Chapter 14:

Unable to repay

When I think of the word "repay," I usually associate it with something of a financial matter, like a bank loan. Sometimes I think of repaying a favor, hence the common phrase "I owe ya one."

What about life? How much does it cost? Can we put a price tag on it? Isn't life far more critical and valuable than money in the bank? Can we repay it by doing a favor? Can we repay it with wealth?

For me, the answer is no.

At one point, I was told my life would soon end unless I underwent surgery. Since then, my physical, emotional, and spiritual lives have been restored and extended.

As I contemplate my journey, I know one thing for sure: countless people made contributions toward saving, restoring, extending, and enhancing my life. I am overwhelmed by the need to repay God and so many people for this new life, as well as the opportunity to share more experiences with my family during my additional time on earth.

> *How can I possibly repay someone for their help saving, restoring, extending, and enhancing my life?*

> *So many impacted my life. How can I change theirs?*

> *How can I try to repay the gift of Life 2.0, knowing I can never entirely do so?*

> *How can I express the emotions I have when I learn that my story has saved another person's life when there are no adequate words available to do so?*

I wanted to express my eternal gratitude to everyone who directly or indirectly contributed to my family and me during my dark moments. This desire is so strong that I began to extend those feelings of appreciation to humanity in general whenever, or wherever, I observe kindness to others.

I feel frustration not being able to find the appropriate words to describe how important it is for me to repay what has been given to my family and me. I am compelled to repay the medical community, the American Heart Association, and God in some way for my gift of extended and enhanced life.

It saddens me to realize there are not enough resources available in this world to even put a dent in the debt I feel I owe for the gift of Life 2.0.

How can I possibly reimburse or provide compensation for what I have received? Repayment in the traditional sense is not possible. I must redefine how I repay humankind and God for the unwarranted blessings so freely and selflessly given to me.

I want to repay those who smiled at me for no reason. It felt good and helped my attitude and positive thinking. I want to reach as many as I can and thank each of them. Each person needs to know they are relevant and valuable and that they contribute to positively impacting and saving lives.

Healthcare workers showed me the power and influence of a kind word, a random act of kindness, and genuine compassion. Why shouldn't I do that for others?

It was then that I felt God's calling for me: live Life 2.0 to the fullest so that others may benefit and prosper in their own lives. His calling compels me to brighten the lives of everyone I can.

If given the opportunity, these are the things I would say to healthcare providers, the American Heart Association, and God.

Healthcare providers and your employees

I can never repay you.

Thank you for allowing me to meet you, a world-class family of amazing people, and thank you for giving my heart a voice.

I have had many opportunities to positively touch the lives of others through speaking, print media, internet, and television. It has been a dream come true to have the chance to thank you and do so as often as I can.

Saving, extending, and rehabilitating lives is extremely difficult and noble work. Your inspiring and instructional approach to helping people like me live on, and live right, so that we may experience these most treasured moments is nothing shy of miraculous. After I shower, the mirror reflects the incision down the middle of my chest and reminds me of the physical correction required to extend my life. It is during those moments that I remind myself how your work continues to illuminate my path and drive me forward.

I am always humbled to be in your presence. You are the unsung heroes for millions of people. Often, I am asked to tell my story. I don't have a story; you do. I was simply a character in one chapter of your great story.

I am here because of you—your planning, organization, and execution. I want to share what you do, why you matter, and the difference you make.

What you do: You make achieving bucket lists possible. Because of you, I have been able to complete my life's bucket list. As a result, I am at peace.

Why you matter: Without you, there is no diagnosis, no surgery, no recovery, i.e., I don't survive. I'm living proof of how much each of you matters. Everyone has a role and contributes. You do this for people who have never been to your facility. I am aware of many accounts of people who heard about my journey, were in a similar situation, decided to get checked out, resulting in the need for life-saving emergency surgery. Your work goes well beyond the walls of your facilities and the patients under your direct care.

The difference you make: The most amazing, precious, and inspirational observation I have is about you. You are just like me; you have the same issues and challenges in life, but you give and give and give and give and ask for nothing in return. You are selfless, and you dedicate your time, energy, and talent to better me. You do what makes Angels smile, and I know this to be true.

You successfully put me on a path to a new life I never imagined possible. God has helped me open my eyes, ears, and heart to a better way to live: a life focused on others instead of myself.

If given a choice between the few short years since I met you or the fifty-seven before, I would take the few short years.

Each of you inspires me: nurses, food services, valets, physician assistants, rehabilitation, administration, physicians, housekeeping, security, lab technicians, operating room staff, and continuing education. Your knowledge, skill, and teamwork gave me confidence. Your encouragement gave me hope. Your attitude and approach to caring practices gave me a life to live.

You placed your lives on hold for me; you taught me about my medications, how to eat, how to exercise, and how to smile for no reason. You taught me how to be kind to a stranger, and I learned how wonderful it feels to be kind. You taught me about the importance of humor in recovery. You encouraged me, challenged me, and even high fived me. Most importantly, you ministered to my wife when I was unable to. My Life 2.0 is built on your example.

Because of your motivation and inspiration, I want to show you how much you matter. I developed a cardio exercise habit seven days per week, along with a diet discipline. I lost fifty pounds, beat diabetes, and maintain excellent vitals to this day. I am eternally grateful, at peace, and loving life as I put into practice the lessons I received from you.

Although I can never repay you in the traditional sense, I will continue to remind you of the extraordinary place you hold in my heart—of your relevance, importance, and value—just as you did for me during my stay and continue to do.

I thank God for all of you in the healthcare industry and will be eternally grateful for the opportunity to have met some of you.

The American Heart Association (AHA)

I can never repay you.

You have been with me the entire way and remain with me today, both showing me how to live better and supporting my passion for helping others.

AHA is a remarkable educator. When I learned I was in danger, I wanted to know what was in store for me, what would happen along my journey. The AHA is the source I used to learn about and understand cardiac catheterization, bypass surgery, recovery, and what to expect overall.

After surgery, I relied on the AHA to help me with living a heart-healthy life. Because of the AHA, I replaced my diet with a disciplined diabetic diet and lost fifty pounds. With that, I learned how to exercise and why that matters so much. Today I maintain a cardio exercise program, which I do twice a day.

The AHA was instrumental in providing tips and ideas for how to live well, resulting in improved blood pressure readings, blood sugar levels, and stress levels for me.

Jim, who I will talk more about later, along with the American Heart Association, has been the perfect partner and source of information for living a healthy life.

Without you, your time, your giving, and the funds you raise, the war being waged on heart disease is over, and unfortunately, we don't win, and people like me don't live.

I'm living proof of how much each of you matters. You see, everyone has a role and contributes to saving, restoring, extending, and enhancing lives. The single most important thing you do is raise awareness, getting the word out about heart disease and how it impacts lives. Increasing awareness helps people have a better chance of achieving their bucket lists and makes a substantial contribution to saving, restoring, extending, and enhancing lives.

I thank God for the American Heart Association and I will be eternally grateful for this great organization and their leadership role in this vicious war on heart disease, the number one killer in the world.

Know this: As survivors, we move on, we move forward, but we never forget. You are never left behind, especially in our prayers.

Thank you, and God bless every one of you.

God

I can never repay You.

I said this prayer moments before surgery, and you answered it.

Please take me today if it is your will to do so. If my life is to be spared, I pray that you will allow me to complete a bucket list I have created for myself. These are the most important things I want to achieve during my remaining years.

#1 Dance with my wife again
#2 Hold hands with my wife and take a walk
#3 Meet my unborn grandchild

Thank You for the life I have lived thus far. I give myself and my fate entirely to You.

I have since accomplished my bucket list.

The dance with June took place in front of over 500 people who are associated with the hospital that provided my care. To recite that prayer to them and to include them in witnessing our dance was a precious moment, never to be forgotten or lost.

We have taken many walks since then. As we walk, I hold June's hand and immerse myself in our togetherness, her touch, and the love between us.

I was able to meet that unborn grandchild. His name is Kevin. Since he is the third, we call him K3 for short. From the moment I was able to hold him and spend time with him, we developed a bond that only God could have made available. God, you listened to me that day and allowed me to not only meet and get to know my unborn grandchild, but You also provided me with a reminder of your presence every time I lay eyes on him.

Answering my prayer and revealing Angels proves to me You are real, heaven is real, and there is far more in store for each of us as we depart this world and come home to You. You have opened my eyes to see there is no such person as a stranger and that You can be seen in the eyes of others, no matter the circumstance.

Because of Your grace, I am no longer afraid of dying. I am at peace and fully inspired to do Your work and pay it forward by positively impacting the lives of others as far-reaching as I possibly can.

God, you made it all happen for my family and me. Your riches have no bounds.

Although Thanksgiving shows up only on every last Thursday of November, I believe a healthcare calendar, if one were to be created, would have Thanksgiving listed every day of the year.

I dream of the day patients can speak to all healthcare providers, workers, and organizations in unison. I imagine they might have this to say:

As patients, we give thanks to each of you. As you care for us

Thank you for putting your life's opportunities and challenges on hold, as you work to better the lives of people like us.

Thank you for sacrificing time with your family and loved ones.

Thank you for your unrelenting effort to keep us comfortable.

Thank you for ministering to our families when we are unable to.

Thank you for the smiles, pats on the back, and high fives.

Thank you for your words and gestures of encouragement.

Thank you for showing your sense of humor.

Thank you for your fast response during emergencies.

Thank you for being a companion.

Thank you for watching over us closely.

Thank you for treating us with dignity and respect.

Thank you for striving to become experts in your field.

Thank you for doing the hard work and dedicating yourselves to providing a gold standard of care.

Thank you for teaching us.

Thank you for lifting each other up and helping your coworker.

Thank you for your teamwork.

Thank you for paving the way for friendship with other patients.

Thank you for instilling in us a sense of worth and value.

Thank you for caring.

Thank you for investing in your education.

Thank you for getting to know us.

Thank you for demonstrating how we can take charge of our recovery.

Thank you for being calm during difficult and stressful times for the benefit of our families and us.

Thank you for your 'round-the-clock beaconing light of hope, compassion, comfort, and love.

As patients, we must move on, we must move forward, but we never forget. You will never be forgotten; you will never be left behind, especially in our prayers.

Thank you for your healing prayers and, when you need it, allowing us to care for you.

With eternal gratitude and love,
Your patients, their families, and their loved ones

Dreams do come true.

If each one of us affirmed one person's value every day, this dream could come true.

Chapter 15:

You are never left behind

I accept that I am unable to repay anyone fully for their contributions to Life 2.0. But I do commit to reminding the hospital organizations and the American Heart Association of the extraordinary place they hold in my heart—their relevance, importance, and value—just as they did for me and continue to do for others every single day.

There came a moment when I knew I had to do more. Whereas the doctors, nurses, and many others in the healthcare system provided me with the medicine I needed to undergo surgery and heal, perhaps June and I could give them the medicine they need for healing as they face difficult challenges every day.

Over time, I made it a priority to remind healthcare providers that, as patients, we never forget. They are never left behind, especially in our prayers.

One day I received a phone call from the hospital asking if June and I would attend their new hire luncheon and give a ten or fifteen minute presentation to the attendees, who were there to celebrate one year on the job. I was honored that the hospital had enough faith and trust that I would be able to enhance a meaningful luncheon. The audience was comprised of both clinical and non-clinical staff.

I began the presentation by describing the set of circumstances that led June and me to that hospital. The main body of the talk centered around how their compassion, smiles, pride, passion, and teamwork gave my family and me great comfort and confidence that everything was going to be okay, that I was okay, and that we would get through my surgery. I emphasized that everyone in that room contributed directly or indirectly to saving, restoring, extending, and enhancing life. Not everyone in the healthcare industry may be directly involved in saving lives, but everyone does participate in enhancing lives, which ultimately can lead to saving and restoring life.

In my career, I have given many presentations. Standing in front of people was not foreign to me. I could tell the presentation was going well, all eyes on June and me, and the only sound in the room was the sound of my voice.

As I usually do when I speak, I scan the audience and make eye contact. I noticed several ladies using a tissue to dry their tears. I asked myself why anyone would cry. I believed I had just told a good news story—nothing to cause sadness.

As the audience began to leave after the luncheon, my talk, and other announcements, I was approached by one of the women whom I had spotted wiping tears from her eye. As she approached me, I noticed her eyes were beginning to tear up again. I extended my hand and thanked her for coming. I then apologized if I hurt her with anything I had said.

"Oh no," she replied. "I was so touched that a patient would recognize our importance, our value. You truly made me feel appreciated, and I desperately needed that. I was meant to be here today listening to you, so thank you and God bless you."

Those tears were the first sign that I can never stop reminding people of their value and importance.

It was in that moment I realized that perhaps June and I had some medicine to dispense. It felt right; it feels as though this is work God wants us to do. In the same way healthcare professionals' care of my family and me positively impacted many people, maybe our caring for others will have an extensive reach. That is what Life 2.0 has taught my heart.

The hospital invited me back several more times to provide the same presentation to each successive new hire class celebration. Life 2.0 inspires me to give back, to express gratitude, appreciation, and love by letting everyone know they matter and they make a difference in someone's life.

Ironically, demonstrating to others that they matter has an impact on me as well. It's like a boomerang. Throw it out there, and it comes right back. By far, the most profound example of this involved people I have never met. I have been made aware of many examples of people who, as a result of hearing about what June and I went through, made arrangements to get themselves checked out. Many received a clean bill of health and were more at peace because of that. I have also learned of situations where the person learned they were in imminent danger just like I was and underwent emergency life-saving surgery. Learning about another life extended because of what my family endured is the most rewarding and fulfilling experience I have ever had.

To experience that impact just one time causes me to view my journey as less scary and horrible. It causes me to see it as cause to give thanks to God for having me and my family go through what we did. Based upon what I know now, if given a choice—undergo risky and significant emergency surgery to repair my heart so that I may live longer or avoid that altogether and keep living as I was—I would choose the operation. I would make that choice because of the impact it has had on others.

Because of the blessings my family received from so many selfless people, I have tried to give back any way I can. Participating in a television commercial and a video story placed on the internet were effective ways of reaching and benefitting others. I looked for other ways to reach out, increase awareness, and express my eternal gratitude, and I found a few opportunities that fit the bill.

Plaque for the hospital

June and I had a plaque made that we presented to the president of the hospital that took us under their care.

Special Recognition Presented to
All Employees of
The Heart Hospital Baylor Plano

As patients in the operation room, our surgeons hold our hearts in their hands and restart them. In the operating room of life, all other clinical and non-clinical employees hold our lives in their hearts and restart them.

Whether we meet or not, you impact, mold, and shape our lives in ways you might not dream possible—physically, emotionally, and spiritually. You teach, you encourage, you challenge, and you give unconditionally, resulting in the most exquisite gift of all—the gift of Life 2.0, which exemplifies the maximum possible patient outcome achievable only by an organization focused on quality at all levels, in all positions.

As patients, we move forward, we move on, but you are never forgotten; you are never left behind. We remember the "little things"—all of them. We think of the employees we have never met, yet they impacted our experience and our lives. Please know that each of you matter; you are relevant and you are remembered, regardless of your role.

We are blessed and honored to have experienced your talents, your compassion, your passion, your Angelic ways, and, above all, your grace. Life 2.0 is a miraculous and inspirational journey, one we praise you and your noble profession for gifting us. We are infinitely thankful for your dedication and endless pursuit to provide world-class gold standard quality care to patients and families.

It is the Angels within you that walk among us, who touch lives and make the "little things" matter. It is our prayer that the Angels will appear in your life and affect you in the same way as when you touched us.

May God eternally bless you,
June and Kevin Kirksey

Homerun for Life event

The Frisco RoughRiders baseball team is a minor league team, and I was selected for their "Homerun for Life" event. I learned that elements of my story would be read over the loudspeaker during a special break in the game, and as my family stood by at home plate, I would run the bases. It was a great evening. My family was there; my surgeon and his wife were there, along with Randy, Marketing Director for the hospital. I love baseball, and although I believed it would be fun to run the bases during the game, I felt awkward because I knew I was delaying the game and keeping these young professional players from playing.

When the time came, we all were escorted to the field. Both teams emptied their dugouts and lined the bases: RoughRiders on first base and the visiting team on third. I had no idea they were going to involve the players. I just knew it couldn't be exciting for a professional athlete in their twenties to see some old guy in his fifties run the bases and keep them from playing. I got the biggest shock of my life, however, because when it was time, I started down the base path, and every single player for the RoughRiders high fived me and said something encouraging and motivating to me.

It was the best feeling ever. I anticipated they would high five me only and say nothing since the crowd couldn't hear them. I was wrong. I heard "way to go" and "you beat it, man," and "grand slam baby," "atta boy," "good work skipper," and on and on. When I got to second base, all I could do was give it up to God. You see, that connection, that bond, that "I understand you and I'm here for you" moment is what I believe inspired my rehabilitation and drives me today.

It's the code of Angels, and they indeed walk among us.

As I round third base, I am met with the opposing team players who all high fived me and also shouted something encouraging to me. I still think about that evening. Those young men did not have to take the extra step and invest in me with their encouragement—but they did anyways.

Cardiac Innovation continuing education event

I had previously spoken at a community health event themed "Managing your risks for heart disease," which was sponsored by the hospital. After that, I was asked to present to the attendees of a continuing education event called "Cardiac Innovations" with my surgeon, Dr. Moore. The event, sponsored by the hospital, helps clinical workers in cardiac healthcare achieve their continuing education requirements. This session represented the first time they would have a former patient come to speak.

I was nervous before the event. The crowd was a large one, and that was coupled with my anxiety to speak alongside Dr. Moore. He kicked the session off, and just as he began, I look around the room and spot the critical care team that was assigned to me during my stay at the hospital. Editha, Brandon, and Beth did so much for my family and me. I could not let them down. My presentation had to be effective. It was in that moment I had an enveloping sense of calm take over, and my anxiety was settled.

I spoke about the circumstances that led me to require surgery and the countless little things I observed that positively impacted and shaped my life.

I also took the time to highlight my surgeon and the type of man he is. I told the audience that if I were to handpick a surgeon, I would pick one who is experienced, has an excellent reputation, and is skilled, smart, and calm. I think most of us would highlight those attributes as necessary. But, if I were to handpick a world-class surgeon, I would add to that list of attributes caring, sincere, supportive, compassionate, gentle, and humble.

Dr. Moore is all of these things.

As I was closing, I looked at Dr. Moore and said, "You did not hurt me like you said you would when we met in your office. You see, you could have never hurt me because you loved my family, provided them with peace, confidence, and comfort, and you brought your best self. I would accept pain and suffering to any degree in exchange for bettering my family, especially in times of need."

Most crucial speech of my life

I had dreamed about having an opportunity to personally thank the entire hospital organization for everything they did for my family and me. I could not imagine how that would be possible until one day I received a phone call asking if I would be the guest speaker at the hospital's annual awards banquet. I was told there would be over 500 people in attendance, and every department in the hospital would be represented.

After I hung up the phone, tears welled up in my eyes and began to run down my face. These were not tears of sadness or happiness; these were tears of utter astonishment and acknowledgment that God was once again working in my life. He is close. I never prayed for the opportunity to address the hospital. I only fantasized about it, hence, I could not say God answered a prayer. What God did do was nudge me once again, demonstrating that I have some unfinished work.

On the evening of the event, June, my son Kevin, and his wife, Jennifer, drove together. As I customarily do, I practiced for what I was planning to say. My anxiety level seemed to be ten times higher than when I spoke at the Cardiac Innovations event.

Racing through my mind was how close I was to accomplishing one of the three bucket list items I asked God to help me with: dance with my wife again. Before we arrived, I asked June if she recalled the first question I ever asked her the day we met.

"Of course, I do," she replies with a smile. "You asked me if I would like to dance."

Much to my surprise, she quickly asks if I remember how she answered. I was not entirely sure my memory was accurate, so I told her she said no. She patted my hand and told me her answer was maybe.

At the hotel where the banquet was being held, we entered a large foyer area that was just outside of the banquet room. The men in suits and women in evening cocktail attire made for a festive atmosphere while everyone was mingling as they waited for the doors to open.

As we enter the banquet room, I stopped in my tracks, in awe of what I saw. Never before had I seen a meeting room this size as immaculately decorated throughout its entirety. The dominant color in the decorations was red; I was not surprised.

After all, it was a heart hospital hosting the event.

As we were directed to the table where we would sit with family and friends, I was shown where I would be speaking. My anxiety was overwhelming. I excused myself from the table, letting June know I needed to go outside and practice my speech. As I left the packed banquet hall, I entered the foyer area, which had even more people than when we arrived. I did not see a quiet space I could go practice.

I stepped into the men's room and began to review my speech. I felt like I was stumbling and forgetting the vital elements of what I had to say. At that time, I put my speech back into my pocket and prayed: "God, You arranged for me to be here tonight. I can't do it alone. Will you please be with me, guide me, and speak through me?" Immediately after speaking with God, I felt calm and relaxed enough to return to the table and wait for my time on stage to deliver what I believed to be the most important speech of my life.

There were several extra-large screens in the room, almost the size of movie theatre screens. For the next ten minutes, video clips of former patients played one after the other. The last video was of me.

Mark Valentine, the hospital president, went to the podium and thanked everyone for coming. After a brief welcome, he invited Dr. Moore to the stage. He then asked June to the stage. June has always had stage fright and does not like public speaking at all. I felt for her as I watched her bravely walk toward the stage with every eye glued to her. About this time, Randy Johnson, the hospital Marketing Director who was seated one table over, caught my attention, reached out to shake my hand, and, with a comforting smile, said, "This is going to be good." I knew it was time. I did not hear much of what Mark said, but when he said my name, all I could do was murmur, "Okay, God. It's Your time on stage."

As I reached the stage, I shook Dr. Moore's hand and gave June a hug. As they took their seats, I stepped up to the microphone. I wanted to take in the sea of people before me, so I slowly scanned the audience from left to right, then began to speak.

What a beautiful group of people! What a great night to celebrate the accomplishments and awards of your colleagues and coworkers and be together and have some fun

It is truly a dream come true to be with you this evening. I have a dream that one day I could share some things I believe you should know. It just goes to show that dreams do come true.

In the video you just saw, I referred to Angels. I am referring to all you, as I have experienced and witnessed your Angelic ways.

If you hear about the guy living Life 2.0, you are most likely hearing about me. Everyone here, whether we have met or not, participated in my recovery and my ability to move forward in life, a life I call Life 2.0., and moving forward is what I would like to speak with you about tonight.

How it started...although I felt fantastic, I had an unusually poor result on a calcium test that I took on a complete whim. That resulted in a date with one of your world-class surgeons, Dr. David Moore. Our date was a blind date, as I did not previously know him, and it certainly was not a date night out on the town. It was half a day in OR #1, just down the street. As I was getting ready for our date, I was physically on borrowed time, mentally beat (I could not fix it), and emotionally panicked. It was just after surgery that we (my wife and family) entered your world. From there, our experience transcended any expectations we had about what was in store for us.

What my family and I experienced from all of you could not have been articulated any better than the sentiments of the former guests you just heard from on these wonderful videos. We all experienced your tenderness, compassion, safety, protection, kindness, humor, smiles, unrelenting care, gentleness, sincerity, humble nature, and, most of all, your grace.

This rich abundance of your kind and giving spirit permeated throughout all lines of business: valet, housekeeping, food service, security, admissions, marketing, continuing education, rehabilitation, and your entire clinical staff of physicians, nurses, aides, lab technicians, and more.

Moving forward, I transformed from a broken to a highly motivated person aimed to show you something, show you the possibility of your work and your ways.

- ***Mentally*** – *I saw you take charge. This gave me confidence and hope. I moved forward making daily choices and taking charge of my health.*
- ***Physically*** – *You showed me how to eat and how to exercise. I moved forward with this knowledge; I lost a lot of weight. I beat diabetes.*
- ***Emotionally*** – *I saw you smile, and I saw you care. You were kind. I moved forward, and every day I try to at least one time express humility and honor others.*

You taught me; you encouraged me; you challenged me. You see, Life 2.0 is not possible without the entire system working in harmony and all lines of business focused on quality. Whether you met me or not, you contribute, and you affect the reputation of the entire system.

As patients, our surgeons hold our hearts in their hands and restart them. You, the hospital of Angels, hold our life in your hearts, and you restart them, you shape them and you mold them in ways I never thought possible— physically, emotionally, spiritually—and then we move forward and onward. So, do you think you matter?

I've been moving forward, and in doing so, I tell others about you. You are acquiring a reputation worthy of your world-class gold standard cardiac care. The number of lives all of you impact is extraordinary and beyond my capacity to completely grasp.

Your goodness is known throughout the world. I have received written prayers for you from people living in London, England, Toronto Ontario Canada, Paris France, Johannesburg South Africa, Amsterdam Netherlands, Melbourne and Sydney Australia, Mexico City Mexico, Kuala Lumpur Malaysia, Bogota Columbia, and countless cities in the United States.

As I move forward, the most important message is not about me; it's about you. As patients, we do move onward, we move forward, but we never forget—nor will I.

I want to tell you what I remember—and will remember for the rest of my life. What I remember most are the little things. Ironically, it is the little things that affect our guest experiences and your reputation the most.

- *I remember the nurse who made my recovery fun by making a guessing game out of testing my blood sugar. It kept my mind off of my chest and the pain. Thank you, Editha.*
- *I remember looking around my room one day when I was by myself, thinking, "Boy, what a clean room, somebody does this, somebody takes pride in this." I remember thinking I would like to meet that person and thank them. One day a gentleman came into the room to clean, and I thanked him.*
- *I remember the compassion at admissions and the young man with a smile the size of the state of Texas.*

- *I remember thinking how exceptional the food was.*
- *I remember the lab tech who made me feel like a king.*
- *I remember my wife telling me how compassionate the security guard and the valet attendant were and how comforted it made me feel that she was being ministered to by them.*
- *I remember the nurse practitioner who removed two tubes in one shot versus one because she sensed how much anxiety I had over this action. Thank you, Terri.*
- *I remember being referred to as Rock Star.*
- *I remember the warm blankets a young lady put on me the day of surgery and thinking how good it felt, and then I thought there must be someone in this place who cleans and stacks these blankets so that this young lady can provide me one. You know, I would like to meet that person one day and thank them. They matter; they make a difference.*
- *I remember the lady behind the desk just outside of the emergency room. She selflessly gifted me with a smile and a wave every morning I attended rehab. You know she did not have to; she just did. I made an effort to go back and introduce myself and thank that women for being the Angel she is.*
- *I remember each exercise physiologist in rehab simply saying, "You are doing well, Kevin."*
- *I remember the chaplain and his gentle ways, Thank you, Rob.*
- *I remember how much I have learned about my heart and cardiovascular system, and everyone is so*

approachable. Goodness, I am sure Dr. Moore is tired of my inquisitiveness. One day I asked him how one sews these small arteries together. Most surgeons, I can imagine, would answer that with "it's magic." My surgeon, Dr. Moore, responded to that with "let me show you" and he proceeds to draw it all out on a piece of paper. I then asked, "Do they ever leak?" to which his reply was "sure they do," and with an astonished look, I asked, "What do you do then?" He smiled and said, "Ya keep on sewing until the leak stops!"

- *I remember the day I was discharged, and as I was wheeled past the nurse's station, I raised my hand and said, "Thank you for saving my life," and the room lit up with smiles and waves.*
- *I remember achieving my first lap around the nurse's station and being rewarded with a high five.*
- *I remember the humor with everyone.*
- *I remember thinking about how supplies and medications I needed always seemed to be available. I remember thinking somebody has to buy these things and make sure they are always here for guests. If you know who this person is, would you please tell me then I said thank you.*
- *I remember leaving the hospital one day while attending an event. There was a man on his hands and knees washing the windows to the door. Just as I said, "You are doing a great job, and I promise not to mess them up," he responded with a gentle smile and said, "It's quite all right if you do, though, sir."*

- *I remember the person in the catheterization lab that broke the ice with me. He could tell how nervous I was and came up to me and said something I promise to not repeat in the presence of Mark Valentine ever again. But, you know, it was by far the most perfect thing to say to me at that moment.*
- *I remember the stranger who stopped and asked if she could help me. Thank you, Carla.*
- *I remember how clean the OR and cath lab are and thinking someone does this, how do they make it so clean? I must be in the right place. I remember this comforted me.*
- *I remember how professional, funny, and accommodating the marketing department, led by Randy Johnson, is. It took me months to obtain one of these "squeezy hearts" (I pull it out of my pocket and show it). If you hear the marketing department complaining that they are missing one, be sure to tell them two things: 1) Tell them you saw it and know where it is; and 2) Tell them it is not coming back!*
- *I remember the incredibly friendly greeting I have always had and seen in the main lobby, not just for me but for others. Thank you, Vicki.*
- *I remember my wife felt I was in good hands and knowing she could go home and rest rather than feel she had to stay at the hospital. Thank you, Brandon.*
- *I remember how your chief executive officer focuses on quality. But, more importantly, how I saw it mirrored*

and mimicked by everyone I came in contact with every line of business. You are doing a good job, Mark.

- *I remember being in your lobby one day, months after my surgery, and an OR nurse walking by, stopping as she looked up at me, smiled, and said with a very warm smile, "I remember you."*
- *I remember learning something about your chief nursing officer. I learned that it is important to her that her staff learn something about their guest which can't be found on their chart. You do a great job, Susan.*
- *I remember the surgeon, my surgeon, who said how "honored, grateful, and privileged he was for the trust and faith I was giving him with my life."*

As patients, we move on, but we never forget, never. I think of you—all of you. I think of you when I get on the treadmill every day, when I order food at a restaurant, when I see someone giving another person a high five, and when I see or hear the word "quality."

You see, I believe everyone deserves an award tonight. You could hear it in the sentiments of the former guests on the videos and in your gift to me enabling Life 2.0. Each of you has a great capacity to affect guests, their families, and their loved ones.

You helped me get up, you helped me take my first step, you loved my family, and you made it possible for me to ask my wife that question again. So the most recent question I asked my wife was on the toll road coming up here tonight. I introduced myself and then asked, "Would you like to dance?"

She said, "Absolutely, yes."

You see, I can't think of a more wonderful thing to do tonight that to be able to dance with my wife in the midst of all of you fine and wonderful people.

My wife and I are blessed and honored to have experienced you and your grace.

I have a dream and a prayer for each of you.

My dream is you move forward and find your own 2.0.

My prayer is that you know the Angels in you are what touch lives and make the "little things" matter.

It is the Angel within my heart, the heart that each of you has touched so profoundly physically, mentally, emotionally, and spiritually, that honors you for allowing me to move on, move forward and wants you to you know that we as patients never forget, you are never forgotten, you are never left behind.

In conclusion, I would like to share with you the very first question I asked my wife thirty-six years ago, after introducing myself. Would you like to dance? I am embarrassed to say I did not win the prize by her saying "yes." She said, "maybe," but after months of work and effort, I won the gold by her saying "yes"—my asking for her hand in marriage.

This question is particularly important to me. As I was wheeled into surgery, I asked God if He were to spare my life to help me achieve a bucket list of the three most essential items in my life. The first item on the list is I want to dance with my wife again. I have a chance, tonight, to achieve that bucket list item.

As I looked toward the table where June was seated with my family and friends, I said:

June Kirksey, just like I did the day we met, I would like to ask you a question. Would you like to dance?

She immediately said, "Yes, I want to dance."

And I closed with:

May God eternally bless each one of you. Thank you.

Kristie

I was determined to follow through on what I said at the awards banquet about wanting to meet the person who cleans and stacks the surgical blankets and thank them.

I learned that Kristie worked behind the scenes in the surgical area. One of Kristie's duties was to wash and fold the blankets that are heated and bring warmth to surgical patients, just as one did for me before surgery. Her job would typically not involve direct patient contact. I will never forget the warmth of those blankets and how I wanted to say thank you to the person responsible for blankets and let them know they made a difference—in my case, a profound difference.

I believe many workers in healthcare do not think of themselves as positively impacting someone's life, let alone saving, restoring, extending, and enhancing one. Even facilities workers most likely never imagine they contributed to life in such a profound manner as I experienced. I wanted Kristie to know the impact of her efforts.

At a pre-arranged day and time, Randy (Marketing Director) escorted me into the surgical area where I met Kristie. I told her about my experiences and how the blanket meant so much for my comfort and peace of mind. I reminded her that even though she may not directly work with patients, she makes a positive impact on them every day. As I hugged her, I noticed tears of appreciation accompanied her smile.

Various letters

Pappas Restaurants: I became acutely aware of the power of acknowledgment, a compliment, and a thank you. I wrote letters to anyone and everyone who impacted my journey. I wrote to Pappas Restaurants. They bought our meal the day before surgery and gave me a t-shirt, such a small gift, but one given with immense love.

Dr. Stack and Kathy: I wrote a letter to Dr. Stack and Kathy and expressed a tremendous amount of appreciation, indebtedness, and praise. I was blessed and honored to have experienced them—their talents, compassion, and passion as they care for their patients.

The heart center: In addition to speaking at their annual holiday party, I wrote them a letter of thanks for being the ones who ignited my journey, which would lead me to Life 2.0.

Dave R Williams: Dave was a builder. His company built our home. I have often heard that most people don't care for their builder after the house is built. In this case, quite the opposite occurred; we became friends with Dave.

One day we received a letter from Dave just before Christmas. He wrote about some of his life lessons. He had cancer and was dying.

Dear Friends:

I have hesitated to share this with you, but I have been encouraged by several people to relate my experiences of the last twenty months. They believe that it may encourage those facing battles of their own.

It seems appropriate at Christmas since my story is one of salvation and redemption. It is what this season is all about.

On New Year's Day, I awoke with the realization that this date represented my fortieth anniversary in the residential construction industry in North Texas. As I reflected on all that time, I began to count my blessings. I had a very successful home building company based in a great community, a wonderful marriage most only dream about, three adult children who I had great relationships with, and two handsome grandsons who were the light of my life.

I had it all.

Ninety days later, I would wake up again. This time at [a cancer center] in Houston where an oncologist told me I had cancer and would need immediate and aggressive chemotherapy. She would offer no opinion as to how long she expected me to live, but I had the sense that it is a matter of weeks.

And, frankly, my prognosis was a matter of days. In my condition, I did not believe my body could sustain life much longer.

I submitted to the treatments. They were horrible. My body began to rebel, and the side effects of the drugs they were relentlessly pumping into my system were taking a devastating toll. I began to decline, and the thoughts of dying were permeating every second of every hour.

During my eight-day stay in Houston, I was rarely alone. Leanne, my kids, and my brother were there for me. Their care was non-stop as I fought to get a footing against a dreaded disease that was winning the struggle for control of my body.

But, one night, I awoke at two in the morning, and nobody was in my hospital room. I had told everyone to please get some rest. So, for the first time, I was alone.

I decided to pray.

Talking to Him was something I was unaccustomed to doing.

There is a balance in the universe. The Earth revolves around the Sun in precise harmony, and the moon revolves around the Earth in perfect balance. There are a ying and yang, there is darkness, and there is light.

Evil is manifested every day in our lives. Poverty, disease, war, intolerance, and hatred are all in the news on a daily, sometimes hourly, basis.

It only makes sense; it only seems natural, that goodness and light, redemption, and salvation balance darkness. I believe evil is counter-balanced by a loving God.

"God," I prayed, "I will only ask you for one thing during this struggle, strength. Give me the strength to fight, and cancer will find in me a formidable foe."

From that very moment, I began to rally. From that very moment, I changed.

God answered my prayer that night in a sterile hospital room surrounded by my fellow cancer patients fighting for their lives.

The next months would be challenging. The chemotherapy would reduce me. From the start, my weight would plummet, and I would lose a total of eighty pounds (OK, OK—I know I NEEDED to lose about forty of that).

But, gradually, I began to improve. Cancer was losing this battle, and I was continuing to get stronger.

I have told some of you that this was obviously among the darkest days of my life. But, strangely, it has brought some of the most uplifting moments as well. I have said things to my wife and children that needed to be said, and my relationships with all of them have strengthened as they supported me in my struggle. I decided that, however bad I would feel, I would continue to work. My involvement has also made a difference—those hours spent doing something productive have aided in my recovery. On countless times, friends uplift me and rally to my side. I have enjoyed seeing my company's employees grow as they compensated admirably for my absence.

So, after twenty months, I have come to a point where I have now allowed myself the luxury of thinking of the future. There have been several pieces of good news from my oncologist over that time, but when she told me that I needed to STOP gaining weight, I knew we had turned a corner!

Since there is no specific medical reason for me to be here, I believe there are only two differences that have made me better.

One is prayer, and the other is perseverance.

There is no substitute for either.

Early on, my friend and associate Gary shared with me a video featuring Stuart Scott of ESPN, who had been fighting cancer for several years. He vocalized something that had been simmering in me.

"I am not here because of anything I have done. I am here because of everything you have done," Stuart said.

Dozens of people have said they have prayed for me. And, dozens of times, I have said, "It is working."

Just before I got sick, a reporter interviews me for a magazine piece. She asked me what I thought was the single thing that has made a difference in my life.

I immediately responded, "I never give up." Perseverance conquers all.

So, now, all my days begin the same way—with prayer and perseverance.

Each day I ask God to continue to give me strength, to continue to heal my body, and to continue to reveal to me how I can make a difference in the lives of those less fortunate.

For perseverance, I repeat every day a speech given to the people of Britain by Winston Churchill at the start of World War II. The Germans were relentlessly bombing London, the cancer of Nazism was spreading across Western Europe, the Americans had not yet joined the fray, and the fall of the British Empire seemed imminent.

Churchill rose and said, "Never give up. Never give up. Never, ever give up."

His words resonate and inspire me each day.

With all the negativity, doubt, and chaos in the news today, I hope my story will uplift you at Christmas.

God is good, hope is alive, and redemption is just a prayer away.

I am living proof.

We do not have the promise of a trouble-free life. Remember, there are no stars without some darkness, and the darker the skies, the brighter the stars.

Merry Christmas to all, and may God bless you as richly as He has blessed me.
And Happy New Year,
Dave R. Williams

Dave was a great man, father, husband, and employer. He left me and others with wisdom about life, which to this day, I try to use. I decided to write a letter to Dave.

Hi Dave

I have written to you a dozen times since you sent your letter over nine months ago, except always in my head. Sometimes I have composed my response while on an airplane, in a hotel room, in the quiet of the evening, and even during the hustle and bustle of everyday life. The difference this time is I am moving it from my heart to paper so I can share it with you. First and foremost, June and I are deeply touched and grateful you are still with us. May God bless you.

I am delighted you wrote about your experiences and sharing them with others. You have deeply touched the lives of others; you certainly did mine. Although you will never forget that precise moment with the oncologist in

Houston, when you experienced the hesitation and lack of affirmation about how much longer you had, I hope to bring you comfort by sharing that I, too, had one of those moments. I understand what it is like to experience hesitation from a medical authority. I understand the fear and what I describe as inner terror and the speed and depth at which the mind attempts to process the shocking and unexpected news. I also understand the ongoing thoughts around our immortality, the ones we knew would come at some point but never expected to arrive when they did. It's like going to hell, but as I prayed for you and heard about your strength and progression, it's like coming back from hell and into the light. You are a great light, Dave, one that shines all around you. You tremendously impact the lives of others when perhaps you don't know how deeply and far-reaching you do.

Although we have not spoken, I have found myself inspired by your story, inspired by the way you think, inspired by you and Leanne and how you two got it right, and this inspiration has helped me be my very best, and in doing so inspire others around me, just because of you. I, too, have had an incredible journey. It is a blessing to have the opportunity to share my story with others. A fascinating realization for me is how we impact others without knowing it and at times, impact those we don't even know. Just two days ago, I had Eddy, your brick mason, over to the house to assess some work I need to have done. I learned about his health challenges and the constant pain he is in with his kidney stones. He is genuinely suffering. During the conversation, I asked if he was still doing business with you; he proudly said: "Yes, sir!" I then asked if he knew how you were doing; he lit up and, with an expression of great pride and happiness, reported you are doing well. The smile on his face and the positivity with which he spoke about you genuinely inspired me, again. Your courage, your strength, your attitude rubbed off on him, overpowered his affliction, and as a result, rubbed off on me in a beautiful way. See how this works? It's fascinating. I tell you this because you are doing it every day, and I wanted to remind you about the power and influence of it all. God did answer your prayer, you were meant to be here for a while longer, you have unfinished business in this world, and I believe it has to do with God using your story to impact and influence others. I want you to consider how far your faith and attitude carry in this world, and when you think you have it, multiply your understanding times 100,000, and then and only then will you be close to grasping the positive magnitude of your story.

You were correct, your story is one of salvation and redemption, and it continues to be so. You alluded to it in your post so I will share with you my conclusion about my experience. But, ironically, it was the best thing that ever happened to me. I see things in this world I never saw before. I see the beauty in everything and everyone around me. I tell people I am living Life 2.0; it is incredible. I also see this in your writings; I understand it, Dave. It's beautiful!

Dave, our paths may be different, but you and I have a shared journey. I had an unusually high amount of calcium build up in my cardiovascular system. It will never go away. That calcium formed levels of blockages that in a very short while would have caused a most probable sudden death. I was meant to be here a while longer. The cardiac specialists tell me I have the highest results from the calcium scan they have seen. I have always dreamed of being #1 at something but never did imagine it would be this. The bottom line is I produce bad things that block arteries and do so rapidly. I got lucky this time but don't know about the future, so you and I share the same journey forward, the passage of the unknown, so let's do everything God wants of us. Everyone on this earth shares that same journey; you and I just happen to have a very profound sense about it.

I am glad you wrote about our living and loving God. Our prayers get answered. God lives, and Angels do walk among us. I have seen them.

I no longer think of you as Dave R. Williams, the construction expert and builder of beautiful homes. I think of you as Dave R. Williams, God's expert mason and builder of a beautiful life, one that is nurtured and fed by an incredibly loving family. You are an inspirational man.

I pray for your continued strength and ministry to so many people in this world who need it.

All the best, Dave. May God's richest blessings be given to you, your family, and your loved ones.
Kevin Kirksey (K2.0)

I am happy I wrote to Dave. He did receive and read my letter, and he passed away not too long after that.

American Airlines: It seems that every time I fly, someone is complaining about something. It could be about the food, the late departure, the ticket price, the employees, the aircraft—the list goes on and on. The airlines can't win with so much negativity and criticism directed at them.

One day, it occurred to me that American Airlines has been blessing my family and me for many years; yet, I have never realized it, nor have I thanked them.

I have never thought about honoring an airline, but why not? I started the letter, addressed to their CEO:

Today I am honoring American Airlines.

You have flown my family and me on every vacation I can remember, and you have done so safely.

Approximately 85 percent of all business trips I have taken, over the past thirty years, have been with your airline, and you have done so safely.

You brought me home the day I received terrible news that my life was in jeopardy. I remember walking to your ticket counter in tears, not knowing if I was going to die that day, die on the plane, or in the parking garage at DFW airport. I remember how kind and gentle the staff at the counter in San Jose was that day.

You flew me on my first trip after recovering from surgery. Not only did you allow me to pre-board (I could walk fine), I remember a flight attendant, without any prompting, literally putting my luggage up for me. I could not lift over five pounds because of the fragile nature of the incision on my chest. What an amazingly giving person she was.

You flew my family on the first vacation we were allowed to take after my recovery. The love and closeness I felt being with my family on our way to our vacation, knowing I was alive and well, was the best of the best feelings I could have.

I find your customer service people to be so helpful, your gate agents to be so kind, and the onboard flight attendants to always be attentive. I have had many fabulous experiences with your airline. I have been with you for a long time and will remain a delighted and loyal customer—and one who tells others about my experiences with you.

I am blessed and honored to have experienced your airline. Although you have endured a lot of changes over the years, you have always had my patronage and will always have it moving forward. I am thankful for your dedication and endless pursuit to provide world-class service to your customers. It is the Angels who walk among us that touch lives and make the "little things" matter. Thank you for all of the little things you do and how you have touched my life throughout my career and my transition to Life 2.0. Thank you for getting me to my meetings, getting me home, and getting my family to our vacations so that I can enjoy my beautiful bride another thirty-four years.

Today I am honoring American Airlines.

Very Truly Yours,
Kevin (K2.0) Kirksey

I believe the business of Life 2.0's focus and priority is how I spend my remaining time in this life doing what I can to better my brothers and sisters. None of them are strangers; they are all friends and family. I can't change the past, but I can change what I choose to do today and tomorrow, for the rest of my life.

Each day I look for opportunities to dispense smiles to people. I look forward to encouraging, complimenting, doing what I can to demonstrate to another person their worth, value, importance, and relevance, just as healthcare workers did when they cared for, healed, and rehabilitated me. It's what God wants me to do.

I remain humbled by all the people who have invested and continue to spend their time, talents, and interest bettering the lives of others through selfless giving.

You are never forgotten; you are never left behind, especially in my prayers.

Chapter 16:

Living Life 2.0 with heart disease

By the grace of God, I am alive today. I believe I know why my story unfolded the way it did. I now live a most miraculous life—one I call Life 2.0—and continue to experience an overwhelming, increasing need and desire to give back, to pay it forward, and to follow my calling.

From my point of view, living with heart disease is multifaceted. Every day I face a physical, emotional, and spiritual component. I am floored by the prevailing nature of heart disease in our world today and how potently it affects the lives of millions of people.

Making a daily choice to live or die has become my foundation for living with cardiovascular disease. If I don't live, I am unable to pay it forward and positively impact the lives of others. As a result, I believe I have a responsibility to do everything I can to maximize the probability of extending my life.

What fuels my motivation is the memory of countless people who met head-on the most threatening aspects of my cardiovascular disease and emotional brokenness, paving the way for me to have more time on earth with my family.

A simple, inexpensive test not only saved my life but was also the catalyst for putting me on a path to a purposeful life.

Physically

I remain a physically broken man; my heart disease is still there. It will never go away, which can be a very sobering fact to accept. I remain "on edge," given I never had a sign or a symptom suggesting something was wrong. At times, I want to hide behind my smile and love for others, but I must move on, move forward, and pay something back.

My daily consumption of medication is meant to help my heart rate, help my blood pressure, and keep the remaining calcium in my heart intact. The best I can hope for is that the calcified plaque deposits in my heart do not break free, form a blood clot, and cause a stroke or cardiac event. The particular medication I take to help keep the plaque intact has deterioration of muscle mass as one of its side effects. Thankfully, the choice between losing muscle mass and dying sooner is an easy one to make.

Every day, seven days a week, I do a cardio workout twice a day—once in the morning and once in the evening. On very few occasions do I miss a workout. I typically only skip one when I am not feeling well. Once I developed this daily habit, I lost fifty pounds and was able to eliminate taking blood sugar medication, which before was necessary to help control my diabetes.

Each workout is short, lasting only twenty to thirty minutes. I like spending half of the workout on a treadmill and the other half on the elliptical while listening to my favorite music. In my early days of establishing an exercise habit, I incorporated games into my routine to facilitate enjoyment and fun instead of viewing exercise as a burden. I would count how many calories I burned at various speeds and inclines on the treadmill and time how long each level took to achieve.

There are a couple of reasons for me to be motivated every day. First, I have a desire to impress my cardiologist each time he orders a stress test for me. It feels good to experience the technician's positive response to how well I performed during the test, as well as the smile on my cardiologist's face during a follow-up visit as he reviews the results with me. He even told me, while chuckling, that these stress tests are not an endurance test, and I am not training for the Olympics. All I could do was reply, "I do it to give back."

My thoughts alone spawn the most motivating aspect of working out. Once the music starts and my workout is underway, I think about why I am doing this and who helped me along the way. I see their faces. I feel their good wishes, their encouragement, and I see the sacrifices they make for humankind. I must remind them of their value by showing them that their contributions are significant and meaningful and do indeed change lives.

Emotionally

There are times I feel sad, afraid, and helpless to do anything about what might happen to me. Will a plaque deposit break free and end my life? Will one of my bypasses fail, causing cardiac arrest? Will this flaw of mine, cardiovascular disease, be the thing that takes me out of this life? I know this: When these emotions appear, I can remind myself that when I am doing everything I possibly can to live, I should not be afraid, saddened, or feeling helpless. I need my family to know how loved they are, and I need others to know they make a difference in this world. I am at peace with dying; therefore, I must continue to listen to God, move forward in life, and focus on investing my energy in making the most positive impact I can. Sometimes I wonder why I even have these emotions, but I suspect they come with being human.

Spiritually

The spirituality of my life brings everything into focus, and it finally makes sense to me.

I think about the Angels who appeared to me on three occasions. Often, during a workout, and when I least expect it, I am enveloped in what I can only imagine is God's presence. The experience is so powerful that it sometimes brings me to tears. Simultaneously, I feel warmth, tingling, comfort, safety, a sense I am cared for, and affirmation while, for a few moments, I experience this omnipotent presence radiating through every cell of my body.

There is no question. I do have a purpose. I have work to do in this life. Experiencing God's presence is like a knocking on life's door, reminding me there is work to be done. I feel a calling, something I never experienced in my life before now. Sometimes when I talk to God, I affirm my understanding of what is going on here. In a somewhat humorous manner, I sense God saying, "I brought you through a dark period and showed you a passage leading to a new and extended life. It's your turn to do something for me."

Somehow, with no words being spoken or heard, I understand my calling.

Even though I am trying to improve myself physically, emotionally, and spiritually, my body won't let me forget the trauma it went through. On occasion, I feel a weird sensation emanating from somewhere in my chest. Sometimes I describe these sensations as little sharp pains, other times they are lingering, aching pains. Early in my recovery, I was convinced these were symptoms of a problem with my heart. But physicians told me the sensations were normal and they were always present—I was just not as in tune with my body as I am now. Regardless of the nature of these reminders, they always send my antennas up, listening for more signs of trouble.

Staying in touch with those who cared for me and being able to acknowledge medical professionals every opportunity I get is excellent medication for my soul. I regularly correspond with my former caregivers and take every opportunity speak to medical professionals and the public. My life is overflowing and rich in blessings. I have so much to be thankful for: my wife, my family, my life, my faith, and all of the wonderful people who impacted my journey to better health.

Life can be a burden for all of us, including things like frustration, doubt, uncertainty, sadness, and anything else that gets in our way and consumes us. As part of living each day with heart disease, I think about ways I can remind healthcare workers of the bigger picture they are part of and the impact of what they do. They are a part of a fabulous system of people who impact and transform lives so that others can further enjoy their loved ones, spend time with friends, and continue to pursue their dreams. So many people played a role in giving my wife and me renewed life together. I pray that all health-care workers realize that even though life presents burdens, they do great work and make such an impact by doing the little things.

I have learned many things since I started living Life 2.0 with heart disease. Just a few key things I've learned include:

The importance of acting on one's health. None of us want to be hypochondriacs, but we should be responsible for our bodies and listen carefully for whispers from God (and, of course, physician recommendations). We can never ask enough questions about our health, and no question is a bad question.

No matter the severity of cardiovascular health issues, there is something available for every patient. I learned to no longer be afraid of being in a situation where I am told nothing can be done for me. The science of treating heart disease and malfunction is the furthest and best it has ever been. I attribute this to the immense amount of research applied in this area along by organizations like The American Heart Association that provide funding to help advance the research.

The importance of forming an exercise habit and making it fun so that a habit can be formed. Make it your own.

The significance of doing little things for others that can monumentally impact their lives. I have come to know that all big things begin with a collection of little things, and the same is true with people and how we treat and acknowledge them.

Each day I sense I am here for a reason. I feel God's calling and Him speaking to me through the lives of others.

Angels do indeed walk among us. I felt them, I sensed them, and I saw them. They are truly present in our lives and this solidified my belief that there is more for us as we depart this earth.

Taking my medications regularly and at consistent times maximizes their effectiveness. Some of them will be a part of my daily regimen for the rest of my life.

Living with heart disease can introduce a friend. What are the odds of two people meeting in cardiac rehabilitation with so much in common? Dan and I share the same birthday, the same outlook on life, the same taste in breakfast foods, and we ended up in the same class at the same time on the same days. I believe it was meant to be. Dan is a very close personal friend. We meet for breakfast every couple of months and have been doing so since our time in cardiac rehabilitation. We look like two average guys having a meal. In some ways, we are. We talk about family, work, life, aspirations, and inspirations, and we relish in the comfort of being with one another. Looking at us, you would not know that we both received the gift of extended life. We met in cardiac rehabilitation class, where we laughed, competed, and eventually formed an incredibly strong, beautiful, and loving bond. I view my friendship with Dan as another one of God's blessings in my life. Dan always puts others first and has led a life working hard for our freedoms and opportunities through his military service. He is a highly decorated man because of his contributions. Not only am I appreciative of his service to humanity, but I am also proud of him and lucky to have him in my life.

So many blessings overshadow the struggles of daily living with heart disease, most prominently the blessing of Life 2.0, which is available to everyone who seeks it. I am humbled, eternally grateful, and awestruck by how miraculous and full of possibilities life can be, and how insignificant living with heart disease has become. I work hard to stay healthy not because I am afraid to die, or because I am not ready for my life to end, but because I want to extend the time I have to learn more about Life 2.0 and to live it the best I can for others.

I would never wish heart disease on anyone. After all, it is currently the world's number one killer. But, perhaps saying that I am deeply grateful for having heart disease is not as odd as it might sound. It led me to the path I am now on—and the journey ahead.

For me, daily living with heart disease is filled with blessings. I did not find Life 2.0; it found me through the actions and love of others. It is a gift, not intended just for me, but for all of humanity. It did not change my life; it gave me purposeful life.

I learn more about it each day that I live and experience others, especially those I have not previously met.

My purpose is to live the example of Life 2.0 for the benefit of others. God has blessed my life in ways that prove His existence and unconditional love for all of us. I have seen Angels in the eyes of others; I have experienced a transformation from a life that was broken to one that is remarkable, amazing, and miraculous. I am so undeserving of these blessings. I can only do what I believe God wants me to do: Live a life focused on others so they might also be introduced to Life 2.0.

Chapter 11:

Nurses – What I want you to know

I do not know when my time on this earth will come to an end. Because of this uncertainty, I do not want to leave without having said what is on my heart for nurses. It is vitally important that I express what I feel in my heart.

All nurses have a special place in my heart, one reserved just for them. They take us into their care when we are at our worst, for example, post-cardiovascular surgery. They work tirelessly and selflessly to care for us, nourish us, teach us, and improve us, and they never ask for anything in return. When we leave their care, we are most likely not fully recovered. They work so hard on our behalf and rarely get to see us at our best. In some ways, this seems unfair, both to them and the patient.

189

I was given an opportunity to express my gratitude and appreciation to those who make a difference to others by writing a letter to the nurses of the hospital, a letter that would be published in the nurse's annual report.

I focused on what they do, how they impact those around them, and how they will never be forgotten.

Moving forward in Life 2.0: Nurses are never forgotten

I believe "little things" make all big things possible. Something very big, I call it Life 2.0, was made possible for me because of the little things nurses did through their caring, compassionate, and giving ways.

In the operating room, our surgeons hold our hearts in their hands and restart them. In the operating room of life, our nurses hold our lives in their hearts and restart, reshape, and mold them in ways you might not imagine possible.

Opening my eyes for the first time as I laid in the hospital room having just had open-heart surgery, I was greeted by the familiar smile, loving words, and gentle touch of my beloved wife, June. Although I was relieved to be alive, I saw fear and despair in her eyes, and then I heard, "Hello Kevin, my name is Brandon, and I will be your nurse today. You are okay; you are fine." He said this with a warm and comforting smile. In just a matter of minutes, I sensed his confidence, experience, knowledge, compassion, and passion for being good at what he does. Even though I had just come from a major surgery, I felt safe around him and under his care. June and I quickly felt at ease, and this turned out to be a tipping point for what would represent an amazing and unforgettable experience with the nursing staff. Honestly, I thought I was just lucky, but as my story unfolded, I learned that I was lucky because the entire nursing organization is world-class.

I will forever remember so many positive things about my experience with the nursing team, mostly little things. My wife, also an RN, told me how comfortable she was with the nursing staff. What a huge relief it was for me to know she did not have to carry yet another burden during a time when I was not able to help her.

Teamwork among the nurses was significantly abundant during my stay. At one time, I needed some extra attention, and before I could blink, several nurses were immediately attending to my issues. They all seemed so highly skilled and highly trained that my helplessness and fear quickly subsided. I recall the wonderful nurse who cared for me in the evening, Editha. She used to play a game with me, which was who could most closely predict my hourly blood sugar test result. What a great way to get my mind off things and give me a little break from the recovery burden I was combating. Another nurse, Beth, one day said "you are my rock star" for taking my first lap around the nurse's station, and that made a profound impact on my recovery. By doing so, she motivated me to work very hard to improve. The nurse who was not even assigned to me, Roy, visited my room to help out during a busy day and stayed a few extra minutes to help me with my breathing, show me how to get up and down, and visit with me for a moment.

One day, while all alone, I decided to get up from the bed on my own. I was unsuccessful. I looked up and saw a nice lady, Carla, someone not even assigned to me, at my door. She entered, and with a smile, she asked, "Do you need some help?"

The nurse practitioner, Terri, made me feel like I was the only patient in the hospital.

Months after surgery, during a visit to the hospital, I saw a team of OR nurses walking through the lobby. One of them came my way, and with a smile, offered a little thing, which to me was huge. She said, "I remember you."

For me, the nursing team was my go-to point for the entire system. I looked to the nurses when I was in pain, when I needed something, when I sought approval, or when I just needed someone to talk to. The nurses were the main cogs in the wheel of my cardiac care—my lifeline. Although there were times when I was alone and the lights in the room were out, somehow, the nurses managed to care for me in such a way that, even then, I felt safe and comfortable.

The nursing team made my family and me feel important and relevant. Every contact with a nurse was, and even today remains, personable. We deeply appreciate each of you for wanting to get to know us and learn something about our life.

Your knowledge, skill, and teamwork gave me confidence. Your encouragement gave me hope. Your attitude and approach to caring practices gave me a life to live. I have often referred to your place of work as the hospital of Angels—my experience with the nursing team and the power of all the little things you do make the Angels smile.

You started something big. I am more than fully restored, living a new and beautiful life, one I did not know existed before you took me into your care. I no longer look for you to enter my room and make it all better because I am no longer hurting or require your nursing care. I am soaring in all aspects of my life, but as I do, I now look for you each day when I invite you into my room of prayer and eternal gratitude. You see, as patients, we move on, we move forward, but we never forget—you are never left behind.

I want every nurse associated with the hospital to know this about me: If I never lived another day, I was blessed to experience what I call Life 2.0, the big thing you started. And for that alone, I have lived a full and rewarding life. Nurses, as guests, we thank you for supporting us, thank you for believing in us, and thank you for caring for us in ways that no one else could.

Because of your work, your beautiful, giving ways, and your relentless pursuit of quality care, I pray the Angels will appear in your life and touch you with the "little things" in the same way you touched me. Thank you for choosing the noble profession you did; I am living proof that what you do matters.

From my innermost self, from the depths of my being, I am eternally grateful and profoundly blessed to have experienced your beautiful, giving ways and benefited from your relentless pursuit of quality care.

Kevin Kirksey
a.k.a. K2.0

Chapter 18:

Family – What I want you to know

*J*ust as I did for nurses, I would like to express what is on my heart for some family members. Perhaps, when I am gone, this can serve as a reminder for them of how dear they are to me and how deeply I loved them.

Pop-pop to K3

I remember when my son and daughter-in-law were discussing what name to give their first child. I was able to name my son after me, so whatever they went with for this child was great by June and me.

The day my son announced that you would carry his name, Kevin, I was beyond thrilled—three Kevins in a row. I was so incredibly touched by their decision, along with being completely surprised. We call you K3.

My third and final bucket list item was accomplished the day you were born. I thank God for answering my prayer. My life is complete.

K3, God reserved an emotion for the time I first laid eyes on you and held you in my arms. There are no words that can describe how connected with you I feel. Your Nana feels the same.

Since that day, you and I have shared a close bond that is very special, very unique, and can never be broken. It came from God, beginning the day I asked for God's help to meet and get to know my unborn grandchild. Not only did God answer my prayer, but He also provided a grandson—you—to Nana and me that we were able to love far more deeply than our most profound imagination could have dreamed.

Please don't be sad or feel bad when I am absent from this world. The absence is only temporary, and until I see you again, I promise to help you along the way and send my love. Pop-pop will always be near; you will feel my presence.

K3, by the time you are old enough to read this book, you and I will have had many beautiful experiences together. When you were a baby, I would talk to you about many things. I would often say, "Any time you need anything, anything at all, just call Pop-pop, and I will be there for you."

I have loved every second of our time together. Whether we are playing, reading, watching videos, wrestling, or just taking it easy, I can't imagine spending my time any better than I do with you.

K3, you have a wondrous life ahead, filled with opportunity and blessings. Sure you will experience disappointments along the way, along with life's everyday challenges and frustrations, but know this: You are not alone. Your Nana and Pop-pop have been there, and so have your mom and dad. Please don't ever feel alone in this world, because you are not. Remember that always.

In case you were curious about your Pop-pop's views on some essential elements in life, I will share them with you here so that you can refer back to them in the event you want to.

Love

Love is your friend. Give it freely with no strings attached. Never ask for it or demand it. As a child, you have shown great empathy for others. That is a very admirable trait to have; it demonstrates you have an immense capacity to love.

Show love through your service. The most excellent example I have of that is your Nana. She always showed her love through her service to her family, friends, loved ones, and even strangers. Your Nana was by your side, and helping your mom, as you were assimilating to the world around you. She watched over you, fed you, bathed you, read to you, and loved you every moment she was with you. Her love for you and the bond you and she have is undeniable and will never be broken. Nana is the epitome of showing love through service. I hope one day you can marry someone just like Nana; your life will be so much better as a result.

Try to forgive others for their wrongdoings. It will happen in your life; we are all human. Forgiveness is a gift for you. When someone offers an apology, try to forgive them. If you can't do that, then, at a minimum, acknowledge them. A thank you goes a long way. Never ignore an apology. That is not a kind thing to do. Always remember that acknowledgment of others is a form of love, a love God gave us all the capacity for.

Family

At the time I am writing this book, Nana and I have been married for thirty-eight years and have known each other for forty. We stayed together regardless of what storms in life came our way. Nana and I invested heavily in our family with our time, our wisdom, and our guidance and made many sacrifices so that the family would be preserved at all costs. Above all things, please do not take for granted anything a family member does for you. Do your best to express your gratitude and appreciation with sincerity.

We loved your dad, our son, more than life itself. I hope and pray that you, too, will enjoy the experience of a family as your haven as we did and have the opportunity to enjoy loving someone as much as we love you.

Friendship

Friendship is like love; it should be given freely without conditions. You may have female and male friends; however, you must have a robust and healthy friendship bond with males. Having a buddy to talk to, to listen to, hang out with, and look out for makes life's challenges far more tolerable. Always be kind to your friends. Kindness and friendship go hand in hand.

Leadership

My dad, your great grandfather, and his dad, your great great grandfather were leaders of men in life. In my profession, because of what my dad taught me, I also rose to a leadership position for the majority of my career.

I became a leader not for me but for my family, which includes you. Your dad, my son, also became a leader of men, also for his family. Suffice to say that it's in your blood. You will become a leader, and just as your great great grandfather, great grandfather, Pop-pop, and dad did, you will empower others to think for themselves, make decisions, and take risks. Your role as a leader is to guide, mentor, and assist others, not to mandate, rule, or impose your will on them. As a leader, surround yourself with people more talented and capable than you. That was the hardest lesson for me to learn in my professional life, but, at the same time, it was the lesson that produced the most significant results.

Throughout your life, take time to smell the roses. Said another way, slow down from time to time, reflect on your life, be kind to yourself, and acknowledge the people and blessings around you. Most of all, pat yourself on the back by recognizing your achievements, big or small. Doing so will positively impact your effectiveness as a leader.

My only regret in life is knowing that you might be in pain one day over my passing. I won't be here to comfort you, but I will in spirit. Please don't feel sad. Be happy that your Pop-pop had a beautiful family for many years, led a fascinating life—Life 2.0—and connected with God, the same God that brought you and I together.

I hope you can find God in your life. He is there, waiting and wanting you to ask for Him. It will be through your relationship with God that you and I will find one another again after my passing.

Pop-pop deeply loves you, little buddy. You are my best friend, my number one guy—always have been and always will be.

When I am gone, if you ever wonder what I am doing, all you have to do is sing the song that I sang to you every day we were together: "Poppy dancing, Poppy dancing, whoo whoo whoo whoo whoo whoo whoo."

That's what I will be doing, thinking of you, with a smile on my face.

Jennifer

Because of you, June and I have received a level of happiness beyond anything we could have ever hoped to receive. I pray that one day, you, too, will experience the same.

We are immensely grateful to you for marrying our son, delivering K3 to this world, and always making an effort to include us.

We have only ever wanted the best for our son. One day you came along. You grabbed his attention, listened to his dreams, became his best friend, and captured his heart. You have unconditionally supported his career, considered his opinions, treated him with dignity and respect, and always stood by him.

From a father's perspective, you are giving Kevin II all that I could ever hope for my son. You are an equal part of our family, a family that has stuck together through every storm and opportunity in life, a family that believes in one another and maintains unconditional love for one another.

Thank you for inspiring my son to be a great husband, a great father, and a great family leader.

I never thought being a grandparent would be so incredibly marvelous. Your son, K3, holds an extraordinary place in my heart, a place that only he can occupy. He and I were bonded the day I asked for God's help in achieving my bucket list. Not only did God come through, but He also presented a young boy who makes this world a better place to live, and who touches the lives of everyone who meets him.

Thank you for being the best mother this boy could ever want. You will never know how appreciative I am for your kindness of allowing him to carry my name, just as your husband does.

It is only natural for a bride's in-laws to be on the outside and less included compared to her family. In our case, you have not allowed that to happen. You have honored us, loved us, supported us, and included us, just as I imagine the daughter I never had would. Thank you for the gift of knowing what it feels like to have a daughter, and thank you for allowing us to continue to love our son and our grandson by making us a part of your family.

We pray you and Kevin II will always honor and respect one another. Keep your arguments and marital fights to a minimum, and do so privately; this will help K3 thrive in the home. One of life's lessons that June and I try to practice is recognizing that being right, or imposing one's will on the other, is never helpful, kind, or important. Getting past disagreement swiftly is the result that matters most.

People often ask us our secret to marriage. My response to that question is to become a student of your spouse. Immerse yourself in their world, even if you initially have no interest. For me, it was shopping. At one point, I did not like to go shopping, and when I did, I wasn't genuinely plugged in to what June was interested in finding, or for that matter what her favorite style was or even her sizes. One day I decided to become a student of hers. I jumped at every chance to go shopping with her, something she loves to do. I made it my business to ask about her thoughts on clothing, shoes, accessories, and almost anything that would help me learn more about her. Over time, I learned. I was able to walk into a store and quickly identify items that were her style and to her liking. Shopping was just an example. Becoming a student of one's spouse and participating in their world, learning their interests and likes, even when you initially might not want to, enhances and strengthens a marriage more than anything I know. We have been married for thirty-eight years, and I look forward to being with her for an eternity.

Thank you for being our daughter, as well as an integral and equal member of our family.

We love you.
Dad II

My son, Kevin II

Kevin Jr.,

You have motivated and inspired me throughout my life. You hold a permanent place in my heart, a place only you can occupy.

For my sixtieth birthday, you surprised me by presenting me with tickets to my all-time favorite band: Tom Petty and the Heartbreakers, section 1, on the floor, close to the stage. For the first time, I enjoyed renting a car because I was with you, and we were taking a road trip together to Oklahoma City for the concert. You treated me to a nice steak dinner before the concert and prepaid for a hotel for us to stay that night so that we could be fresh for our drive back. I was beyond elated for having the opportunity for this father-son time, on the road, doing something together, and just spending life together. You take after me in the "busy" department—working tirelessly at your job while having a newborn son to deal with—yet you stopped and took time out of your life to spend some quality time together. It doesn't get any better.

The first book I ever wrote, ***There Is No Other,*** was written for you from a place of immense love. It only had three chapters and took me thirty-two years to write.

- Chapter 1: The Interview
- Chapter 2: The Advice
- Chapter 3: My Prayer for You

I carefully thought out each chapter and constructed them in such a way that they would pass the test of time while strengthening in value.

Chapter 1: The Interview

Throughout my life, I often wondered what it would be like when I looked in the mirror and said, "You have now reached Grandpa stage." Frankly, I prefer the Pop-pop stage. Would it be a time when I come face to face with the harsh reality that most of my life is now over and behind me? Would it be a time I get down to the business of truly reflecting on my mortality? The truth is, it is nothing like what I thought. The most important thing that hit me was an overwhelming sense of pride in you, Kevin, for achieving the status of fatherhood. Not every man gets here, not every man survives here, but every man who enters has the opportunity of their life, an opportunity that only God himself can provide. Welcome, you have arrived! Be vigilant and observant of the world and the forces all around you. You have a young one to love, to protect, to provide for, and to guide throughout his life as best you can.

Fathers know things about their sons, things sons don't realize we know. Kevin, I know what it was like to have me as a dad. I

204 | *Life* 2.0

came to see the impact on you, both negative and positive, of the decisions and choices I made in my life. I know your struggles as you grew: personal, academic, social, emotional, and spiritual. I knew when I had to rescue you, and I knew when I had to hold back so that you could save yourself. Balancing that is extremely difficult for a father to do. You will experience this yourself with K3 one day.

I decided there was one more job I had to do as you take the reins. I had to send you into fatherhood with the best possible start and tell you some things you need to know. I decided to give you the book as a Christmas gift I had been making for approximately 11,680 days (thirty-two years).

There is no better time then now, as you enter fatherhood, for me to tell you some things you need to know.

The day K3 was born, October 1, 2016, I looked at you in the hospital room and thought it felt like I had just passed the baton to you. Profoundly, it felt like my job was complete; it felt like you had the reins to take it from here. As I looked at you, with a smile on my face, I decided that I had one last job to do: to send you into fatherhood knowing what you mean to me. You began the most important job you will ever have in your life, and I want you to have the best start possible.

Now is a time for me to tell you some things you need to know.

"There is no other" is the phrase that permeates my thoughts when I think of you, Kevin. You must know how deeply you have motivated and inspired me throughout your life and how you occupy a permanent place in my heart, a place only a son can fill.

I decided it would be best to write it down because the written word lives forever, and the day is coming when I won't be on this earth to show and tell you about the things you are about to read. I want you to have something to hold on to, should you find comfort in doing so.

What would I want you to know? There is too much to put on a piece of paper. Hence, I will stick with the important ones. For me, the important ones are those things that would surface if I were to be interviewed by God and the topic was you.

What follows is an excerpt of what my responses sound like in an interview with God, answering essential and personal questions about your role in my life.

It might start with God saying, "So, Kevin, tell me about your son." Then He listens.

I would respond, "That's a great question, God. I am so happy you asked. Let me tell you about my son, Kevin."

There is no other guy I would rather see happy in life.

There is no other I would rather play ball with.

There is no other guy I would rather have silly fun with.

There is no other I would rather watch dance with my bride.

There is no other guy I would rather be in Maui with.

There is no other I would rather hang out with, just doing anything, talking about anything, especially those deeply intellectual and philosophical talks we were notorious for having.

There is no other I would rather see happy in life.

There is no other I would rather go to a baseball game with.

There is no other I would rather see enjoying his friends.

There is no other I would rather coach, or watch coach.

There is no other I would rather listen to speak at the Meyerson Symphony Center—or any venue for that matter.

There is no other I would rather see enjoying their loving grandparents.

There is no other I would rather watch hit a home run, or throw a guy out at first base from deep into left field, or be on the mound striking out the opposing team's cleanup hitter.

There is no other I would rather watch play volleyball and deliver a kill shot, block an outside hitter, or make a perfect pass.

There is no other I would rather play golf with.

There is no other I would rather see hit three three-pointers in a row in a basketball game, as I murmur, "That's my boy."

There is no other I would rather see enjoying and drawing comfort from his four-legged pal.

There is no other I would rather see smile the smile of accomplishment from getting their first job, getting that first paycheck, or getting that next great job.

There is no other I would rather support educational pursuits for and be there applauding as he earns his college diploma.

There is no other I would rather share a Thanksgiving, a Christmas, or any day with.

There is no other I would rather see, standing tall, beaming with love, as he anticipates joining hands and marrying.

There is no other I would rather protect and sacrifice my life doing so.

There is no other, as you can see by now, that would motivate me to work as hard as I can to pave the way for opportunities abundant in his life.

There is no other I would have in my family and call son.

There is no other I would rather father a grandson for his mom and me.

God, that's my son, Kevin. Thank you for asking me to tell you about him.

Chapter 2: The Advice

Kevin, I have known for a long time this day would arrive: the day my role would change. I no longer have you to raise, but, rather, I have you to love, support, and observe with pride as you begin to be a parent, just as I did thirty-two years ago.

As we both assume new roles, I would like to share my advice for you, dad to dad, followed by sharing my prayer for you.

Please know I have complete faith in your ability to succeed at anything you set your mind to doing. Mom and I raised you to be courageous, thoughtful, confident, and focused. The advice I offer originates from my own life experiences and is meant to assist and guide you, both as a father and a man, during the journey that lies ahead.

Do not overextend yourself. There will be many interruptions competing for your time and attention. Remember that you can only give 100 percent of your effort, so, learn to say no and choose wisely how you spend your time.

Do not put too much pressure on yourself. Tension and stress will mask the love and support that Jennifer and K3 must have for your family to be happy, and that happiness will give K3 a solid foundation for becoming the man I know you want him to be. Stress is an archenemy to your family unit; revoke it. Learn to acknowledge it, learn to laugh at it, but master it quickly and render it powerless against you and your family. As a husband and father, this should be a priority.

Take time during your journey to stop and smell the roses. Doing this could mean taking a walk in the middle of your busy day or leaving work early to attend one of K3's functions. Sons especially need their father's approval and will look for you when you least know it. Whatever his interests are, be there for him. He will be looking for you. Investing yourself in this way will fuel you and make your life, including your marriage and parenting, much improved and vastly more effective. It's important.

Treat every person you meet as an individual, and demand of yourself that you always do so with kindness, dignity, and respect. We are all God's children. Do for His children as you would want others to do for yours.

The primary benefactor of the advice so far is your son, your wife, your loved ones, and your friends.

This final piece is just for you. Society and many of the people in your daily life will bombard you with their thoughts, ideas, and wishes for how you should think, live, and interact with others. Sometimes this is a good thing—but not always. The values and morals we raised you with will be challenged in distinct ways, sometimes subtle ways. You will no doubt have to make many decisions as you navigate forward in life. We trust that you will make wise ones, ones that reflect who you are as a person. Do not be influenced to mimic the ways others think or do things. Use your head and decide for yourself, work to live, and become the conductor of the orchestra of your life.

Chapter 3: My Prayer for You

Kevin, at times, I wish I had a redo as a father, a husband, and a friend to others. I have grown to recognize the choices I should have made, but shamefully did not. I have come to know that God exposes a father's mistakes and shortcomings to his sons so they can be the ones with the opportunity to make better choices and decisions—to surpass their fathers. Truthfully, Kevin, that is what we want of our sons: to surpass us in every way. It gives us the sense that maybe we did something right. Many fathers would express this as wanting their sons to receive a better education, a better job, or even earn more money. I understand and agree with these things, and I pray you do those as well. There are things, however, which will set you apart and cause you to soar and surpass those before you. It is these things that are in my prayer for you.

The following is what I pray you will treasure and hold in the highest regard as you navigate through the choices and priorities in your life.

I pray you unconditionally love and respect your wife and your son. Tell them every day how you love them, how you enjoy them, how nice they make you feel. There will be times you won't feel like it…Do it anyway.

I pray you never raise a hand to your wife or your son. If they raise a hand to you, turn and walk away. Don't argue in front of your son; it will poison him.

I pray for you to speak with your wife every day. Confide in her, no matter how bad, how silly, how embarrassing, how uncomfortable the discussion may appear to be. Encourage her to do the same. You will find the purest love, love you could never imagine, makes itself available to you. This type of love is a gift from God.

I pray for you to become a student of your wife and your son. Think of them as the teachers and you as the student. After all, is there anyone more qualified to teach you about your wife than your wife? Is there anyone more qualified to show you what your son is all about than your son? Learn what they like, what their passions and dreams are, what they want from you. Be willing and able to immerse yourself in their world, and do so with a smile. That could mean reading books you don't care for, or shopping at places you would not go yourself, or learning some activity for the first time even though you have no interest in it. Show up for them; be present, be interested, and demonstrate you care about them. The possibilities are endless. Your wife craves this; your new son needs this from you. You will discover your marital bond becomes stronger than before, your connections more meaningful, and your wife and son will become even more fascinating!

After sixty years, I have come to deeply understand that our family, our relationships, and how we treat those we meet are all that matter—and those things are all we have.

Perhaps years from now, you too will experience the warmth, the love, and the respect for your son as I have for you. I trust you will be nodding your head in affirmation, accompanied by a smile, as you too write your legacy to your son and pass on the wisdom you acquired from the beautiful gift we call life.

Most importantly, I pray for you to continue to strengthen your relationship with God and come to understand what God's grace is all about. There is work here. There is study as well, but there are great riches for you and your family. Kevin, His angels walk among us. I have seen them. He is the only path to salvation. He lives!

Lastly, I pray for you to understand that no matter where you are in life, no matter what situation you find yourself in, no matter what age you are, your mom and I will forever love you and will forever be with you.

I give eternal thanks to both your mom and God for the gift they gave me: the gift of you as my son.

I could not have been prouder of you as you were growing up. You never knew how much I boasted about you at work, how many times I brought you into my presentations to customers, my meetings with colleagues, lunches, dinners with friends, and even presentations to the public at large. Over the years, so many people you do not know knew you through me. I estimate I have heard over 5,000 times, "How's Kevin doing?" or "How's that boy of yours?" I can't express how proud I am of your athletic achievement, your academic achievement, and your career achievement. I am super happy that you became a great speaker, a confident man, a resourceful man, and one who works very hard to achieve. You made me proud, Kevin. I don't know how God did it, but He built you precisely how I would wish for my son.

You are now simultaneously working the two most significant, most challenging, and, by far, most important jobs you will ever have on this earth: husband and father. The rewards of these jobs, if done right, will far surpass the summation of all rewards you could ever tally up in a lifetime.

So, here we are, young man. You surely recall me running around the house, or the Kea Lani, shouting, "Is there no one else?" as I mocked Brad Pitt in the famous fight scene from the movie *Troy*. I recall the fun and laughter we all had with that. I certainly hope your mom does not ever release the video. Let's keep that a family secret, okay?

Let there be no mistake or question about a father's love for his son—most importantly, mine for you—just as you will experience with your son.

Love,
Dad
a.k.a. K1, Poppy, Beve, Bevo, Big Guy, Mo, Big Boy, Pop-pop

My wife, June

My dearest June,

There is not enough time in this life to properly and fully profess the love I have for you. There is not enough paper in the world to accommodate the words needed to offer a description of what you truly mean to me.

Let me begin with an apology. I am sorry for the mistakes I made as a husband and as a father and the terrible and frightening experience you endured as a result of my health issues. If I could take it all back and do things over, I would. However, the journey we took together, and the storms we endured along the way, made our bond what it is today—the most miraculous union of two people I could ever have imagined.

With regards to marriage, I am saddened when I hear about the misfortune that some couples experience when they grow apart, fall out of love, and lose the fight to keep their bond together by growing and thriving as one.

I give you all of the credit for making sure that did not happen with us. You have taught me, and allowed me to truly experience, patience, kindness, fairness, forgiveness, and, above all, grace. You are my best friend, my eternal love, and my only.

You are like a blue diamond: rare, legendary, and forever holding immense value for those who know you. You are a blessing to everyone you come in contact with; I am profoundly proud to be your eternal life partner.

I love you more today than I did yesterday. That has been true every day for the past forty years.

If a book were ever to be written about how you express your love, it would contain chapters on sacrifice, loyalty, service, voice of reason, humor, kindness, and respect.

I love you for the sacrifices you have made. You are a college-educated woman who pursued a degree in nursing. After working as a registered nurse in the hospital, you were promoted to Director of Admitting. Your career was in full swing, and when our son was born, you sacrificed your job for the good of our son. I recall how important it was for you to be with him and to be able to nurture him as he was growing up. You applied this level of commitment and sacrifice to our marriage and family unit, always putting your interest in us ahead of your own.

I love you for remaining loyal to me, our family, our pets, our friends, and our grandson—not once did your love waiver for those you cared about the most.

I love you for the way you show your love. The phrase "actions speak louder than words" must have been developed to describe you. You show your love, appreciation, kindness, and caring through your service to everyone around you. It is not enough for you to hold hands and say "I love you" over and over; it was always necessary to for you to show your love in ways that never required you to say, "I love you." Your demonstration of service manifests itself daily in how you present yourself, keep things around you clean and organized, support my career and travels, and make sure everyone is well-fed in a healthy manner. You have always been okay with doing what others wanted to do, even though it may not have been your first choice. You are the epitome of the phrase "actions speak louder than words."

I love you for being my voice of reason. In our life together, I have been the impulsive one, the one to react to any situation and hit it head-on. You, on the other hand, were always there to be my voice of reason, to show me an alternative way to look at solving any problem. You taught me, by your example, how it was best to never confront another person with anger, frustration, or an elevated voice, even if they made a mistake that was costly to us, and even if they were in the wrong. You were the only one who could hold me back and reason with me about what the appropriate response or action might be in any situation. Thank you.

I love you for being a great example of being kind and respectful. I have seen you hold doors open for people when it should have been the other way around, demonstrating how a small act of kindness can result in delighting another person. Many times, I witnessed you conversing with or just saying "hello, how are you" to others far less fortunate. By spending time, even for a moment, with strangers, you validated their value and gave them a touch of warmth in their hearts. You bring them life. When someone made a mistake, you never made them feel bad or guilty; you were always kind and gentle with them.

I love you for your humor. You have always been the consummate comedian. You can walk into a room and within minutes bring everyone present to laughter. You have proven this to be true with family, friends, and strangers. Humor is something good for the soul, and you have used it to impact the lives of others positively.

I love that you never give up. I believe you are the example of what God intended for each of us in a marital bond. We have suffered the roughest of storms a marriage can face, but we always managed a find a way past them. I attribute the success of our marriage to you. Often, I felt I was 10 percent of the man I should have been in a marriage. I always saw love for me in your eyes, and although I have been undeserving of it, you held us together with your steadfast belief and unwavering commitment to me, our marriage, and our family.

In the introduction of this book, I referred to my life at that time like the calm before the storm. Because of you, and only you, we are enjoying the calm after the storms in our life. By us holding together, no matter the situation or circumstance, we are now engulfed in love far more magnificent and a bond far stronger than we could have ever imagined possible. Because of you, I finally get it. I am at a loss for how to properly thank you for everything you have done to ensure we arrived at this place of receiving God's riches.

As I look back at our lives together, perhaps we experienced God's best lesson on marriage. We fought and battled the demons that wanted us to lose and go our separate ways. We have won that battle and find ourselves in a place of rest, happiness, love, peace, and togetherness as one: the calm after the storm.

You are my love, my life, my happiness, my peace, my everything. I want you to also know you are today, always have been, and always will be the most beautiful, sexy, smart, funny, and loving woman in the universe. I look forward to spending eternity as one with you.

Flanking both sides of our home are two stone pillars with lanterns for lighting the path to enter our home. On those pillars is a plaque with the words "Chateau de Grace," meaning home of grace. The world needs to know that you are grace, the one who our home was named after and who fills this home with love.

Thank you, God, for watching over our marriage. I love you, June, more than anything or anyone in this world. I would lay down my life for you.

I will love you, cherish you, and be with you for an eternity,
Kevin
a.k.a. Beve

Chapter 19:

Readers – What I want you to know

Through my experiences, I have learned that Life 2.0 is a journey, a process that builds upon itself over time. It is not an overnight sensation. It takes time, focus, and energy to open my heart to a world where there are no strangers each day. The more I can view life through the eyes of others, the more profound my understanding about life becomes, and the more it brings focus on what God wants me to do.

I believe Life 2.0 is available to everyone. It does not discriminate by age, gender, race, or nationality. I also do not think it takes a life-altering experience for it to awaken in our hearts. How I learned—center stage of a life-threatening circumstance, followed by lifesaving surgery—is not a pre-requisite for finding and embracing Life 2.0. For me, it started with a simple question to another person, opening the doorway to this new life. Open-heart surgery was just the vehicle that transported me to a place in life where I would begin to see, hear, and feel living in a more meaningful and profound way.

Observing the actions of others and the little things people do were the keys to a change in my thinking about the people around me and the life I am living. As I watch and listen for the little things, the goodness in others surfaces, and my understanding that there are no strangers in this world deepens. During my stay in the hospital, my wife and I experience many selfless little things handed out by others. They are not asked to do these things; they just did them out of the kindness of their hearts. Their giving ways opened my heart to a new way to live—Life 2.0 was born.

For some time, from surgery through the completion of rehabilitation, Life 2.0 manifested through the healthcare providers I was surrounded by, both clinical and non-clinical. Their selfless ways, their dedication to helping humanity, even though they have their own life battles to fight, inspires me to consider all people in the world around me in the very same way.

In the hospital, my life was affirmed daily as valuable, meaningful, and relevant. It made me consider that perhaps this affirmation was a lesson on how I should live my life. I am inspired to do the same for people in the world around me, regardless of who they are, where they are from, or anything about them, and not ask for anything in return. It demonstrates their worth—their value.

It started with little things, such as offering a smile to a stranger, holding a door open for someone, giving a compliment, or having a brief conversation with someone and letting them know they are essential to their families, their loved ones, and this world. I began to witness something I had not before understood. It was almost as if they came alive.

Could it be possible that affirming others and reminding them of their value, importance, and relevance can breathe life into them?

My conclusion is yes.

Affirmation and expressing gratitude for others is a form of love that we all can give. People respond to love.

Once I realized there are no strangers in this world, only brothers and sisters, I was able to look at someone and recognize they are just like me. We all have to deal with life's afflictions. When I see someone I have never met, I wonder what burdens them. Job loss? Betrayal? Grief? Health issue? The list goes on and on. I believe our brothers and sisters all need a ray of light in their lives, something that soothes the sting of everyday living. That ray of light originates in Life 2.0—a way of life each of us can live.

The perspective that no one is a stranger reminds me of how similar we all are and helps me more genuinely affirm others. Doing so can positively impact people well beyond those I come in direct contact with, another one of the profound lessons I have learned. I am reminded of times when someone I had never met learned about my medical situation, got checked out, and also had their life saved from a severe condition that would have killed them. I think of the hospital employee who had little patient contact and had a former patient seek them out and thank them for doing an excellent job. We never know how our actions may change the lives of others. What I do know is that each of us can reach and impact the lives of people we have never met.

I learned I had to try and be the best I can be—physically, emotionally, and spiritually—and be my best for another human being, something that also benefitted me personally. I became surrounded by peace and had no reason to fear death, no reason to be stressed, and no reason to be anything other than a positive influence on others. Sure, this sounds like a life of panacea; it is not. We are all human beings, and nobody is perfect. We all make mistakes; we all have our demons, and we all exercise poor judgment. I believe God wants me to mend my heart and become closer to Him by focusing on positively impacting the lives of others. Life 2.0 comes from the heart, a heart that is open and welcoming to all people from all walks of life, one that recognizes all people as brothers and sisters rather than strangers.

Angels do indeed walk among us. For me, they revealed themselves through the eyes of others. I interpreted this as a sign that the life I should be living, Life 2.0, can be found deeply rooted in the eyes and lives of others. I have experienced nothing as powerful, loving, peaceful, nurturing, and reassuring as what the Angels gifted to me in a matter of seconds.

Living a life where I can choose to work hard at focusing on others instead of myself is far more rewarding and fulfilling than I could have dreamed possible.

Life 2.0…it comes from the heart.

My hope, wish, and prayer for anyone reading this book is that you consider how different, new, and fulfilling life can become by simply changing focus toward others, realizing we all genuinely know and understand one another and there is no such thing as a stranger. By considering this approach to living, you will find that you, too, can breathe life into others with simple, straightforward, and genuine affirmation of another's value, importance, and relevance through the little things you do. These little things will make lasting impressions and most will influence others to do the same. Your efforts and actions will extend well beyond what you can imagine. I believe that is what God wants from all of us.

I am eternally grateful for God, my wife, my family, and all people. We are all in this together, and we all know something about each other, regardless of whether we have met. I am profoundly humbled by God's presence and grace and for the revelation of Life 2.0.

God bless you,
K2.0

About the Author

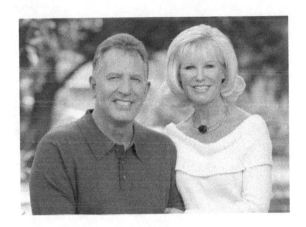

*K*evin Kirksey has lived, and documented, his story of profound transformation to living Life 2.0. Kevin's journey, including the unusual set of circumstances that led to his extended and enhanced life, has been shared with many through writing, speaking, print media, internet, and television. Kevin works with healthcare organizations and the American Heart Association to raise awareness of cardiac disease so that lives can be saved, restored, extended, and enhanced. Kevin and his family reside in Dallas, Texas.

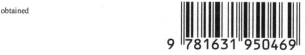